S0-EWH-169

AIDS

Problems and Prospects

WITHDRAWN
WRIGHT STATE UNIVERSITY LIBRARIES

Adapted from **Hospital Practice**

Illustrated by **Ilil Arbel** *and* **Alan D. Iselin**

Designed by **Jack Meserole**

AIDS
Problems and Prospects

Edited by

Lawrence Corey, M.D.

Professor of Laboratory Medicine, Microbiology, and Medicine
Head, Virology Division
University of Washington School of Medicine
Seattle, Washington

A HOSPITAL PRACTICE BOOK

Published by

Norton Medical Books

W · W · Norton & Company
New York · London

WRIGHT STATE UNIVERSITY
FORDHAM HEALTH SCIENCES LIBRARY

Copyright © 1993, 1992, 1991, 1990 HP Publishing Co., New York, N.Y.
All rights reserved
Printed in Hong Kong by South China Printing Co. (1988) Ltd.
First Edition

ISBN: 0-393-71015-7
W. W. Norton & Company, Inc., 500 Fifth Avenue, New York, NY 10110
W. W. Norton & Company, Ltd., 10 Coptic Street, London WC1A 1PU

Illustration Credits:
Ilil Arbel: Chap. 2/Figs. 1–3
Alan D. Iselin: Chap. 1/Figs. 1–4; Chap. 4/Fig. 1.

Notice: Our knowledge in clinical sciences is constantly changing. As new information becomes available, changes in treatment and in the use of drugs become necessary. The authors and the publisher of this volume have taken care to make certain that the doses of drugs and schedules of treatment are correct and compatible with the standards generally accepted at the time of publication. The reader is advised to consult carefully the instruction and information material included in the package insert of each drug or therapeutic agent before administration. This advice is especially important when using new or infrequently used drugs.

1 2 3 4 5 6 7 8 9 0

Contents

6 The Prospects for AIDS Vaccines 85
WAYNE C. KOFF
National Institute of Allergy and Infectious Diseases

7 HIV Infection in Maternal and Pediatric Patients 97
CATHERINE M. WILFERT *Duke University*

8 Reducing Occupational Risk of HIV Infection 115
JULIE LOUISE GERBERDING
University of California, San Francisco

9 Partner Notification for HIV Control 131
FRANKLYN N. JUDSON *Denver Public Health*

10 AIDS, Activism, and Ethics 145
DAVID J. ROTHMAN *and* HAROLD EDGAR
Columbia University

Index 157

Contributors

LAWRENCE COREY, M.D.
Professor of Laboratory Medicine, Microbiology, and Medicine
Head, Virology Division
University of Washington School of Medicine
Seattle, Washington

HAROLD EDGAR
Julius Silver Professor of Law, Science, and Technology
Columbia University School of Law
New York, New York

JUDITH FEINBERG
Assistant Professor, Department of Medicine
Division of Infectious Diseases
Johns Hopkins University School of Medicine
Baltimore, Maryland

JULIE LOUISE GERBERDING
Assistant Professor of Medicine
University of California, San Francisco, School of Medicine
Director of the HIV Prevention Service
San Francisco General Hospital
San Francisco, California

PHILIP GREENBERG
Professor of Medicine and Immunology
University of Washington School of Medicine
Member, Fred Hutchinson Cancer Research Center
Seattle, Washington

KING K. HOLMES
Professor of Medicine
Adjunct Professor of Epidemiology and Microbiology
Director, Center for AIDS and Sexually Transmitted Diseases
University of Washington School of Medicine
Seattle, Washington

DANIEL F. HOTH, JR.
Director, Division of AIDS
National Institute of Allergy and Infectious Diseases
Bethesda, Maryland

FRANKLYN N. JUDSON
Director, Denver Public Health
Chief of Infectious Diseases, Denver General Hospital
Professor of Medicine and Preventive Medicine
University of Colorado School of Medicine
Denver, Colorado

WAYNE C. KOFF
Chief, Vaccine Research and Development Branch
Division of AIDS
National Institute of Allergy and Infectious Diseases
Rockville, Maryland

JAY A. LEVY
Professor, Department of Medicine
Research Associate, Cancer Research Institute
University of California, San Francisco, School of Medicine
San Francisco, California

MAUREEN W. MYERS
Assistant Director, Treatment Research Program
Division of AIDS
National Institute of Allergy and Infectious Diseases
Bethesda, Maryland

DAVID J. ROTHMAN
Bernard Schoenberg Professor of Social Medicine
Director, Center for the Study of Society and Medicine
Columbia University College of Physicians and Surgeons
New York, New York

DANIEL S. STEIN
Medical Officer, Medical Branch
Division of AIDS
National Institute of Allergy and Infectious Diseases
Bethesda, Maryland

CATHERINE M. WILFERT
Professor of Pediatrics and Microbiology
Chief, Pediatric Infectious Diseases
Duke University Medical Center
Durham, North Carolina

Introduction

This monograph on HIV infection and AIDS is based on a series of articles that appeared in the journal *Hospital Practice*. The response to this series, along with its timeliness, has motivated the decision to update and publish the material in book form.

HIV infection has become part of mainstream medicine in most coastal cities of the United States, and indeed in much of the world. Its continued spread in North America indicates that the affected population will constitute an integral factor in medical care delivery, rural and urban, coastal and inland.

The pace of scientific research and the social, political, and health care changes associated with the recognition of the AIDS epidemic have been extraordinary. Although progress in many of these areas has not been quick or sustained enough to satisfy many communities, most notably those most devastated by the epidemic, the fact is that there has never been a health care issue that has evoked such a massive scientific and political response.

HIV infection has placed our national and international research and health care systems under unprecedented public scrutiny. The complexity of the issues, and of the syndrome that underlies them, has created a new subspecialty of medicine, "AIDSology," as well as a plethora of new journals and textbooks devoted to HIV infection. Indeed, this pattern of specialization may in itself be a part of the problem we now confront. Our ability to recognize the infection and its manifestations, the understanding of its pathogenesis and progression, and basic counseling for patients and families must all be integrated into the mainstream of medicine.

It is our intent that this text will elucidate current concepts of HIV infection in the context of the sentinel issues that form its background and provide practitioners with a short review of current management strategies. As the second decade of the AIDS epidemic starts, a retrospective and prospective overview of what has been learned and what must be learned to achieve control of this infection seems appropriate.

LAWRENCE COREY, M.D

Seattle
August 1992.

1 The Retroviruses and Pathogenesis of HIV Infection

JAY A. LEVY *University of California, San Francisco*

The time lapse between human immunodeficiency virus infection and the clinical manifestation of severe immune deficiency was one of the conceptual stumbling blocks that delayed acceptance of HIV as the etiologic agent of AIDS and its prodromal manifestations. This lag ranges from months to 10 or more years. However, retrovirus infections with similar manifestations are not unknown to animal virologists. HIV has been classified as a member of a subfamily of retroviruses—the lentiviruses, a group that includes the simian immunodeficiency virus, the visna virus of sheep, the feline immunodeficiency virus, and the equine infectious anemia virus.

These viruses have several features in common: a long incubation period (hence the term lentiviruses), tropism for hematopoietic and nervous system tissues, and an association with immune suppression. Each of the lentiviruses has a variety of pathologic effects, but in general, only one effect is prominent for the cited viruses in a given species. In sheep, it is neurologic disease, and in horses, an autoimmune hemolytic anemia. In humans, primates, and cats, immune deficiency is the common clinical manifestation, but some individuals have succumbed to HIV infection showing only neurologic disease or primarily bowel disease, with apparently normal immune systems, at least by conventional criteria.

Two genetically distinct forms of HIV have been isolated from patients with AIDS. HIV-1 is the type associated with the disease in central Africa, Europe, the United States, and most other parts of the world. HIV-2 has been found primarily in infected persons visiting or living in western Africa. However, it is also spreading. HIV-2 has the same tropism for cells of the immune system as HIV-1 and causes similar disease, but it has more nucleotide and amino acid sequence homology with the simian immunodeficiency virus than with HIV-1. The primary nucleotide sequence of HIV-2 differs by about 55% from HIV-1. There is, however, enough cross-reactivity with HIV-1 proteins to detect most cases of HIV-2 infection by the ELISA test for HIV-1 used in blood banks; 10% of HIV-2 cases might be missed. The following discussion primarily concerns HIV-1, but it is also generally relevant to HIV-2.

In morphology and structure, HIV closely resembles other lentiviruses. HIV is an envelope virus, so-called because it has a lipoprotein coat similar to a cell membrane, which surrounds a cylindrical core containing the viral RNA genome. The envelope bears transmembrane spikes of a 41-kDa glycoprotein (gp41), each spike being associated with a knob of a 120-kDa glycoprotein (gp120) (Figure 1).

Envelope viruses usually infect by fusing with the membrane of target cells, either on the cell surface or in endocytic pits. HIV seems to fuse on the cell surface. To undergo fusion, the virus presumably needs to attach to the cell by a receptor. Because lymphocytes and macrophages are the cells primarily infected by HIV, investigators considered the CD4

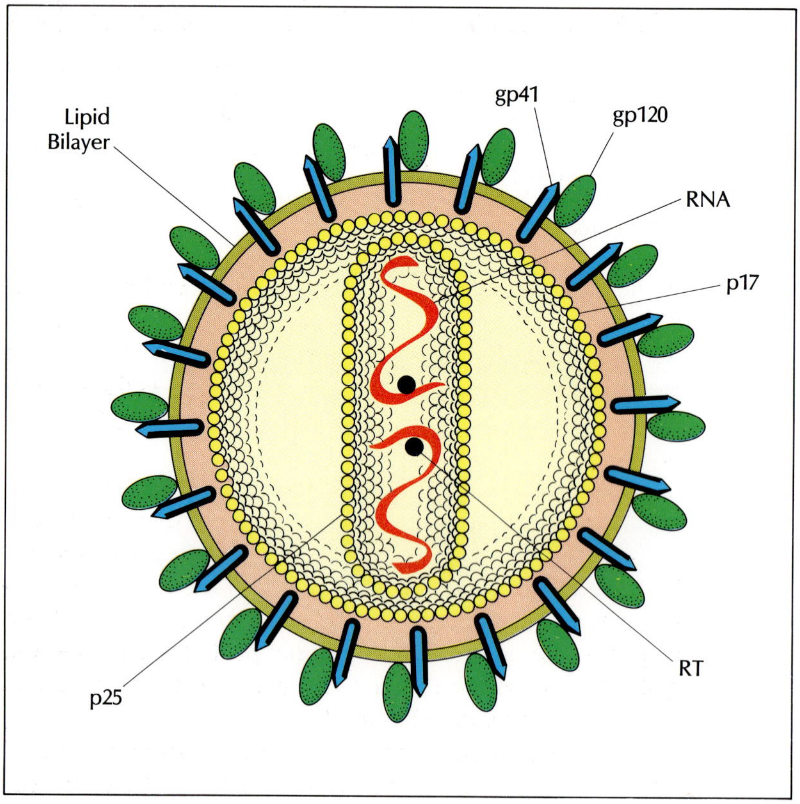

Figure 1 HIV has a two-layered lipoprotein envelope that surrounds a cylindrical core containing the viral RNA genome. Reverse transcriptase (RT) is closely associated with the RNA. The core protein p25 forms the cylindrical shape of the nucleoid. Glycoprotein complexes stud the surface with transmembrane spikes of gp41 protruding from the envelope, each being associated with gp120. The core protein p17 forms the matrix of the virion particle.

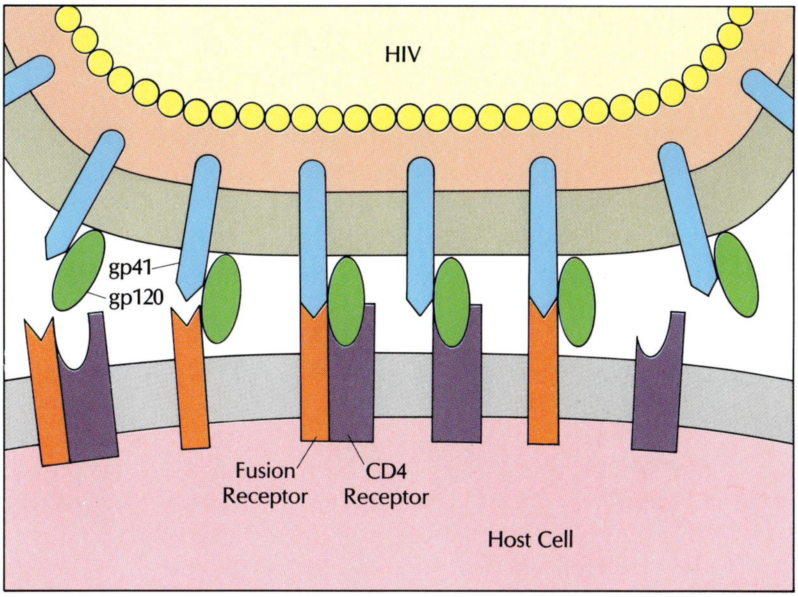

Figure 2 HIV infection may involve a two-step mechanism of attachment and fusion. Attachment may be effected by binding of viral gp120 to the CD4 surface molecule on some T cells, B cells, and macrophages. Virion fusion has been postulated to occur by a specific interaction between another viral protein—perhaps gp41—and an as yet unidentified cell surface receptor that may mediate such fusion. Either receptor might bring about HIV infection, but the most efficient virus entry would be via both receptors.

molecule—a marker on the surface of helper T cells, B cells, and macrophages—the most likely receptor, and indeed, it was quickly shown that the virus does bind to CD4. However, it is now clear that not all cells that express CD4 are infected by HIV, and some cells that lack the marker, such as astrocytes, skin fibroblasts, and bowel epithelial cells, can be infected, although less readily.

The inconsistency of CD4 binding suggested that the molecule merely provides an attachment for the virus and a second step is necessary for fusion. Some human T cells that express high surface levels of CD4, for instance, cannot be infected by HIV. Many envelope viruses do require two steps for infectivity—attachment and fusion. We believe that fusion requires contact between a distinct part of the viral envelope, probably gp41, and a specific region of the cell membrane, which we hypothesize is the fusion receptor (Figure 2).

It seems plausible that fusion without attachment could occur if the virus comes in contact with the fusion site, but attachment may facilitate virus entry, perhaps by inducing a conformational change in the viral coat that brings the fusion portion of the envelope closer to the cell membrane. Alternatively, cells that lack CD4 but are nevertheless infected by HIV may have an entirely different receptor for the virus. That possibility is being investigated.

The role of the CD4 receptor in mediating HIV infection has important implications; blocking this viral receptor could potentially prevent infection. Soluble CD4 has been synthesized and shown to bind and neutralize free HIV virus in vitro. The finding has generated considerable interest in the possibility of using recombinant soluble CD4 as therapy for AIDS, but such an approach presents some problems. For one thing, the CD4 receptor on the helper T cell is also involved in self-recognition and antigen recognition. This makes the receptor essential in the immune system both for prevention of autoimmune reactivity and for most cell-mediated immune responses. Furthermore, CD4 probably is not the only receptor for HIV. Thus, before soluble CD4 is considered for therapy, it must be shown to be both noninterrupting to normal immune function and, if not universal, at least dominant in its antiviral effect.

When the virus enters a cell, it uncoats and, in the manner of all retroviruses, transcribes its RNA genome into DNA, which integrates into the genome of the cell. Assembly of progeny virions takes place in the cytoplasm and at the cell membrane. The newly formed virions can spread to other cells after budding from the host cell into the extracellular environment (Figure 3). Or they can spread by fusion of the infected host cell

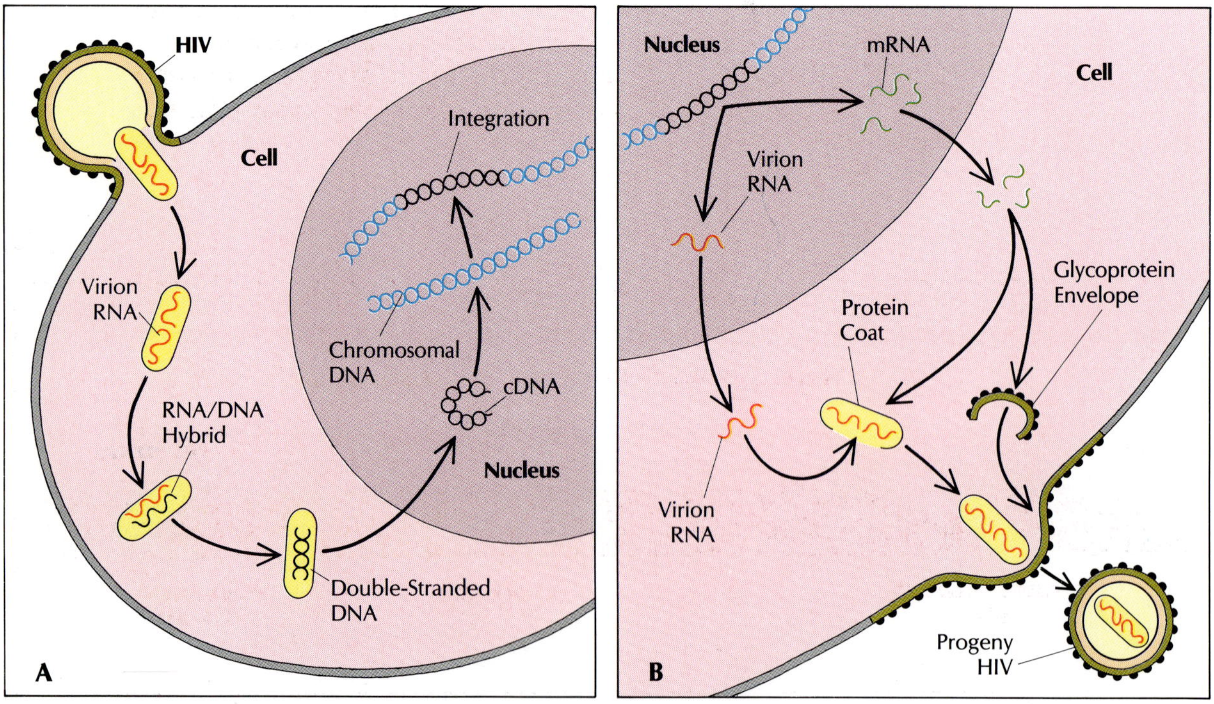

Figure 3 When HIV has fused with the cell membrane (A), the virus uncoats, bringing its core into the cytoplasm, where its reverse transcriptase initiates events that lead to production of RNA-DNA hybrids, double-stranded DNA, and finally circular but noncovalently bound cDNA copies of the viral RNA genome. The cDNA goes to the nucleus and integrates into cellular chromosomal DNA, where it may remain latent, producing little viral protein or RNA. Or, when the host cell is activated (B), viral cDNA produces mRNA, which codes for proteins necessary for virus replication and viral particles and virion RNA, which is the viral genome. The genome is packaged into infectious particles at the membrane and leaves the cell by budding, as shown, or by a poorly defined cell fusion process.

membrane with the membrane of an uninfected cell. This process of virus production may kill the cell, depending on the viral strain and cells involved.

HIV can apparently also remain latent within the cell in an integrated, proviral state, producing little messenger or viral RNA. In the latent state, the provirus may not induce antibody formation, because HIV proteins are not expressed, and thus not recognized by the immune system. Nevertheless, viral DNA has been detected in infected white blood cells by the polymerase chain reaction technique, which amplifies small amounts of DNA. The incidence of latency as the end point of HIV infection is unknown but probably rare. It has been demonstrated in a few individuals who did not seroconvert for up to three years, and perhaps in two others who went from seropositive to seronegative. In many people, both latently and productively infected cells can be found in the blood. Most infected people make antibodies to HIV even if they are asymptomatic, and they remain seropositive.

The need for effective therapy, especially a vaccine against AIDS, has spurred efforts to clone the HIV genome and determine functions of its coding units. One approach is to eliminate a gene and observe the effect on the virus in culture lymphoid cells. Such experiments show that each of the virus's three major structural coding units (*gag*, *pol*, and *env*) is essential. If any is eliminated, the virus falls apart. As we shall see, genes appear to have effects that can increase or decrease virus production (Figure 4).

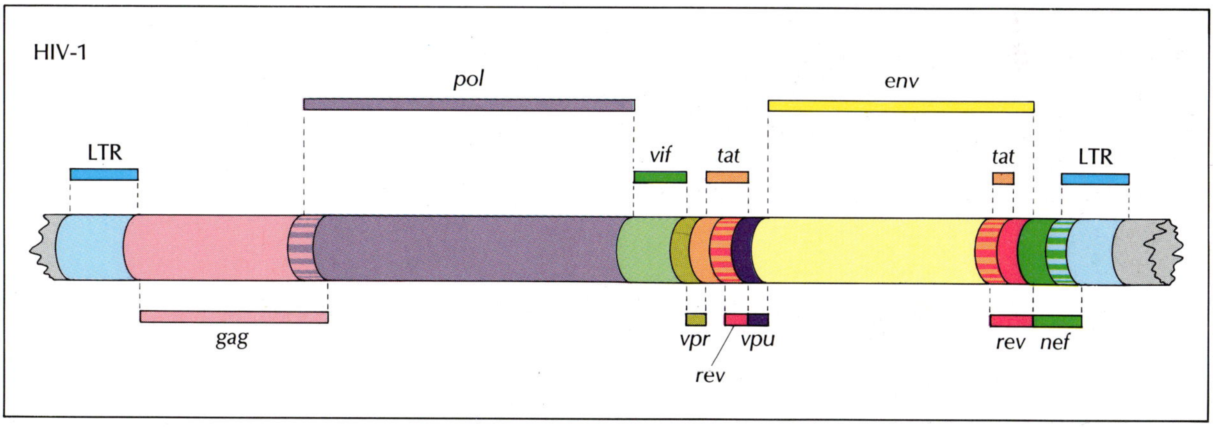

Figure 4 In common with other retroviruses, the HIV genome has three structural genes: *gag* and *env*, which code for proteins that form the viral core and envelope, respectively, and *pol*, which codes for reverse transcriptase and other enzymes that catalyze transcription and tailor the core and envelope proteins. Three regulatory genes—*tat*, *rev*, and *nef*—code for proteins that can enhance (*tat* and *rev*) or inhibit (*nef*) virus replication. Three remaining genes—*vif*, *vpr*, and *vpu*—code for viral infectivity factor, viral protein r, and viral protein u, which appear to influence HIV infectivity. Long terminal repeats (LTRs) contain sequences that help initiate and control replication. Regions that have major overlapping sequences coding for different HIV proteins are indicated.

The HIV Genome

The *gag* sequence is one of the first that is transcribed. It is called *gag*, for group-specific antigen, because one of its products is a protein common to all viruses. The *gag* sequence codes for proteins that form the core, or nucleus, of the virus. The *pol* sequence codes for the polymerase that enables transcription of viral RNA into a DNA copy, as well as integrase (which helps integrate viral DNA into host cell DNA) and a protease (which cuts the proteins coded by *gag* and *pol* into active forms). The *env* region genes code for glycoproteins that form the exterior, or envelope, of the mature virion. The major known products of these genes are two aforementioned highly antigenic glycoproteins known as gp41 and gp120.

For simple retroviruses, structural genes are all that is needed for replication, but the lentiviruses, including HIV, have added regulatory or accessory genes. By the process of elimination, scientists have found that some regulatory genes enhance HIV replication, others impede it. The genes that enhance replication are *tat* (transactivator), *rev* (regulator of expression of virus), and *vif* (viral infectivity factor). The *vif* region product appears to be responsible for maturation of viral proteins at the time the virion buds from the host cell.

In contrast, the *nef* gene (negative factor) seems to suppress virus replication. Eliminating this gene, instead of paralyzing the virus, actually enhances its replication. It may inhibit synthesis or transcription of the viral genome after HIV infects a cell. We suspect that the *nef* gene is responsible for the state of latent proviral integration into the cellular genome described earlier. Several other regulatory genes have been identified, but their function remains unclear. HIV-1 and HIV-2 differ with respect to the nucleotide sequences of at least one of these genes; the *vpu* gene is unique to HIV-1, the *vpx* gene to HIV-2. However, the replicative cycles of both subtypes are similar.

Modes of Transmission

Inoculation of selected cells with HIV in tissue culture usually results in a productive infection, although the levels of virus replication and cytopathology vary considerably from one viral isolate to another, as well as with the cell type infected. Replication of HIV to high titers in cultured CD4+ helper T cells often produces a characteristic cytopathology: the formation of multinucleated giant cells and balloon degeneration of the cells (Figure 5). However, productive infection of T cells seems to require T-cell activation.

The multinucleated cells represent multiple fused cells (syncytia). Ballooning appears to be due to increased permeability of the cell membrane, which permits an influx of sodium, potassium, and calcium ions with water. In cell culture, as the virus spreads by cell fusion, cell death

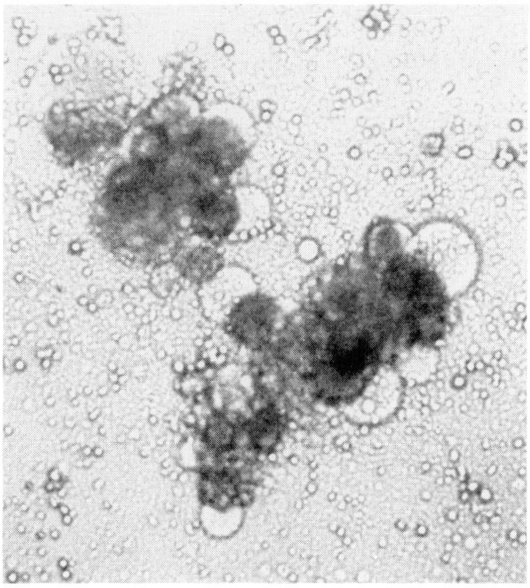

Figure 5 HIV replication in white blood cells can cause them to fuse and form multinucleated giant cells. Infected cells eventually balloon and degenerate. Ballooning is thought to result from increased membrane permeability with consequent influx of electrolytes and water.

usually ensues, and eventually most of the cells in the culture are killed. However, productive HIV infections of cultured cells, including helper-T-cell lines, are not invariably cytopathic or lethal. Infection of cell cultures can proceed without formation of syncytia or cell death. In vivo, viral spread by cell fusion could theoretically proceed indefinitely, whether or not the virus is cytopathic.

The concept that the virus may remain latent also has serious implications, because unlike viruses that destroy the cells they replicate in, HIV can apparently lock itself into the chromosomes of the cell. Because the virus does not synthesize protein in the latent state, it is not recognized by the immune system. It could spread in a somewhat surreptitious manner to other, uninfected cells, to many different tissues, and perhaps via a latently infected cell from one host to another.

Even when the virus is actively replicating, cellular transmission is most likely the dominant form of HIV spread. Studies in our laboratory have shown that the level of *cell-free* virus in body fluids is relatively low, compared with the number of infected cells (Table 1). Thus, unless the infected cell is destroyed, it could transmit the virus from one person to another via blood or genital fluids. In attempts to develop a vaccine against HIV, the role of the infected cell in transmitting the disease is a matter of some concern. Vaccines that prevent free virus transmission may not be sufficient to prevent HIV infection.

Strain Differences

Within each of the two subtypes of HIV, multiple strains have been identified. In our laboratory, we have found more than 1,000 different strains of HIV-1. Whereas each infected individual appears to have only

Table 1. HIV Isolation from Cell-Free Body Fluids and Body Fluid Cells: Results from the Author's Laboratory

	Isolations/Attempts	*Estimated Quantity*
Fluid		
Plasma/serum	45/46	10–1,000 infectious particles (IP)/ml*
Tears	2/5	<1 IP/ml
Ear secretions	1/8	5–10 IP/ml
Saliva	3/55	<1 IP/ml
Urine	1/5	<1 IP/ml
Vaginal or cervical	6/16	<1 IP/ml
Semen	5/15	10–50 IP/ml
Milk	1/5	<1 IP/ml
Cerebrospinal fluid	21/40	10–1,000 IP/ml
Cells		
Peripheral blood mononuclear cells	89/92	0.001%–1.0% of infected cells
Saliva	4/11	<0.01%
Bronchial fluid	3/24	Unknown
Vaginal or cervical fluid	7/16	Unknown
Semen	11/28	0.01%–5.0%

*For comparison, note that for hepatitis B infection, particle counts may range from 10^6 to 10^9 IP/ml.

one predominant HIV-1 strain, some patients from Africa have shown the presence of HIV-1 and HIV-2 simultaneously in their blood. The remarkable heterogeneity of HIV-1 was first recognized when it was discovered that viral isolates from different patients had differing responses to the same neutralizing antiserum. Some isolates are readily neutralized by serum from many different HIV-infected patients, others are not. Other features that distinguish HIV strain include differences in ability to infect, replicate in, and kill a variety of cell types in vitro (Table 2).

Table 2. Viral Characteristics Defining the Heterogeneity of HIV

Cell tropism	Sensitivity to serum neutralization
Replication efficiency	Sensitivity to serum enhancement
Cytopathology	Restriction enzyme sensitivity
CD4 antigen modulation	Genome sequence variation
Latency	

Virulence

Generally, the genetic differences among isolates are relatively minor, but they may influence biologic and pathologic behavior of the virus. Nucleotide sequence diversity is common in the *env* gene and appears to account for the varying susceptibility of different isolates to serum neutralization. Neutralization is believed to be mediated primarily by the interaction of serum antibodies with envelope gp120. Genetic differences in HIV strains may be reflected as well in the cell type infected, how quickly and how well the virus replicates, and whether it is strongly or weakly cytopathic or noncytopathic.

In our laboratory we observed that the most virulent HIV strains are isolated from patients with advanced disease, whereas strains isolated from seropositive subjects without symptoms infect weakly and replicate slowly in cell culture. In view of the progressive nature of the disease, this raises the question of whether a relatively nonpathogenic strain can become more virulent over time.

Comparison of biologic and serologic characteristics of the viruses isolated from the same HIV-seropositive subjects at different times suggests that the virus does undergo changes that contribute to virulence. For instance, the HIV-1 strain originally isolated from a patient with oral candidiasis replicated less efficiently and was less cytopathic than the HIV-1 strain isolated five months later, when the patient had *Pneumocystis carinii* pneumonia and Kaposi sarcoma. Partial gene sequencing of the two viral strains indicated that they were closely related and substantially different genetically from strains isolated from other HIV-infected patients.

Viral heterogeneity may account for the differing pathologic expression of AIDS, i.e., for the fact that some patients have primarily neurologic disease, some primarily bowel disease, and some primarily immunologic disease. The virus infecting an individual may determine organ pathology. In patients with AIDS dementia, the macrophage is the primary cell infected in the brain; in vitro, HIV strains isolated from the brains of AIDS patients with neurologic disease replicate best in macrophages. The same isolates replicate in T cells, but they are not cytopathic to T cells. This finding could account for the relatively normal T-cell counts observed in some HIV-infected patients with neurologic disease. Viral isolates from the brain are also less susceptible to antibody neutralization than isolates obtained from the blood of the same subjects.

These observations suggest that HIV evolves over time, acquiring a phenotype that allows it to replicate efficiently and become cytopathic in a specific cell type or target organ. To date, research has focused on HIV tropism for cells of bone marrow origin, and particularly on the CD4+ helper T cell and the macrophage, but the virus may have the potential to infect a great variety of cell types. As noted earlier, HIV has been either cultured or detected in a number of cell types not derived from bone marrow, including glial cells and astrocytes in the brain, skin fibroblasts, and bowel epithelial cells.

Latency

Viral latency may be another factor related to pathogenicity. Very little is known about latency except that the *nef* gene seems to induce a state of latent HIV infection or low replication in cell culture—because if the gene is eliminated, replication proceeds at a higher level. Cecilia Cheng-Mayer in our laboratory has found evidence that the gene may in some way contribute to or be associated with the emergence of the more virulent phenotype. She transfected the *nef* gene into cultured T cells (which then transcribed the gene product) and found that HIV replication was suppressed in cultures inoculated with HIV from asymptomatic HIV-seropositive subjects, but not in cultures inoculated with virus from patients with advanced AIDS.

The finding suggested that HIV strains recovered from symptomatic patients are resistant to *nef*. The product of the *nef* gene is a protein with properties involved in certain intracellular activating signals, but it is unclear whether *nef* acts on the cell or on the virus or whether its function is altered or lost over time. Current research is aimed at answering these questions.

Host Response

This discussion has focused so far on what the virus does to the host, but there is another side to the pathology of HIV: what the host does against the virus. In some infected individuals, the two effector limbs of the immune system can be diametrically opposed in their response to HIV. The humoral immune system hyperresponds to infection, whereas cell-mediated immunity seems to gradually fail. Polyclonal, almost indiscriminate B-cell proliferation proceeds in an uncontrolled manner as platelet, neutrophil, and T-cell populations decline. High levels of serum antibody are characteristic of the early stage of the disease, but most of the antibodies are directed against antigens previously present (such as herpesvirus) or against normal tissue antigens. Indeed, autoimmunity can develop, as evidenced by thrombocytopenia, neutropenia, and lymphopenia, as well as peripheral neuropathy.

Neutralizing antibodies are, of course, beneficial, since they halt spread of the virus in the host, but many infected patients fail to produce such antibodies to their own HIV strain. If antibody is not neutralizing, it may either have no effect on the virus or actually enhance its spread. Enhancing antibody has been detected in several HIV-infected patients. It forms antigen-antibody complexes with the virus via the Fab receptor on the antibody. Attachment to a cell via the Fc receptor or complement receptor may then allow the virus to infect cells that do not express the CD4 receptor.

Enhancement is a troublesome concept because it suggests that the virus may be able to subvert the antibody response to its advantage. Enhancing antibodies increase in titer over the course of HIV infection. They are expressed in vivo more readily in the later stages than in the early stages of the disease.

The failure of the cellular immune response remains one of the major puzzles of AIDS. HIV exhibits little cytopathology early in the disease, yet a decline in the CD4+ T-cell population is a hallmark in later stages of the disease. Many reasons can be given for the phenomenon: autoimmune destruction of T cells, nonspecific killing of CD4+ helper T cells by cytotoxic CD8+ cells, natural killer cell destruction of lymphocytes expressing viral antigens, and low-level cytopathology (particularly in stem cells) that over time depletes the white cell population. All of these effects have been demonstrated in vitro, and it is assumed that they could occur in vivo.

Virus replication seems to be a major factor in disease progression. During the initial, acute, phase of HIV infection, the viral core antigen p25 and infectious virus can be readily detected in the blood. Later, the virus and antigen disappear or decrease substantially, and a resistant state seems to develop. In those who subsequently progress to AIDS, the antigenemia reappears, reflecting virus production. In addition, a reduction in antibodies to the core protein is noted. A sudden decline in the CD4+ cell population often marks the clinical onset of AIDS.

CD8+ T Cells

HIV-seropositive subjects who maintain a resistant state can remain asymptomatic for long periods of time—sometimes more than 10 to 12 years. Studies in our laboratory indicate that another aspect of cell-mediated immunity—one mediated by the CD8+ T cell—is responsible for keeping the virus in check. These cells have been shown to be as cytotoxic to HIV-infected cells in culture as they are known to be for cells infected with any other virus.

Nevertheless, HIV-seropositive subjects, even asymptomatic long-term survivors, always harbor the virus in the body, even when evidence of HIV cannot be found in standard culture assays of peripheral blood cells. This observation suggested two possible explanations. Either their CD8+ cells had killed any virus-infected cell present in the blood or the cells were preventing the virus from replicating.

The second possibility proved to be the case. When the CD8+ cells were removed from the blood cell cultures, HIV replicated in the remaining cells, and when the CD8+ cells were returned to the cultures, the virus disappeared. Thus, in addition to the previously noted cytotoxic effect, some CD8+ cells have a suppressing effect on HIV that keeps the virus in check without killing the cell. The effect is distinct from the function of the CD8+ suppressor cell in classic immunology: suppression of B-cell proliferation and antibody production.

This CD8+ suppressing effect on HIV replication most likely is not unique to that virus. Similar effects have been described with suppression of replication of Epstein-Barr virus, cytomegalovirus, herpes simplex, and probably other viruses that the human body harbors over long periods of time.

Very few CD8+ cells are needed to suppress HIV replication in an asymptomatic subject—a ratio of about one CD8+ cell to 10 CD4+ cells in vitro is sufficient—but as the disease progresses, the ratio reverses. The number of CD8+ cells is not the important factor, because this cell population may actually increase as the disease advances, but the antiviral activity of the cells diminishes.

We believe that HIV suppression is the function of a subgroup of CD8+ cells. These cells may be responsible for production of a cytokine with antiviral activity. Christopher Walker in our group has obtained evidence for such a soluble factor by placing CD8+ cells from HIV-seropositive subjects in the bottom chamber of a well, separated by a filter from CD4+ cells replicating the virus in the top chamber. The factor passes through the filter and suppresses the virus in the cells at the top. Efforts are under way to characterize and synthesize the factor because it seems to offer a natural approach to controlling the virus.

As we have seen, HIV is heterogeneous with respect to properties associated with virulence in the host. Some strains cause disease rapidly; apparently more common are strains that emerge over time with pathogenic features. In order to change into a virulent form, the virus has to replicate. It appears that as long as the host's immune system can suppress the virus, it will remain relatively nonpathogenic. An important question is whether a breakdown in antiviral activity eventually occurs or whether a pathogenic strain evolves and finally emerges to destroy the immune system. The two possibilities are, of course, not mutually exclusive, and we still cannot define the phenomena involved. What is clear is that HIV infection sets in action an ongoing fight between the virus and the host's immune system. Anything that disturbs immune function may advance the disease. Thus, while discussion of chemotherapeutic approaches to HIV infection and AIDS is not within the scope of this review, from an immunopathologic view it should be noted that the indiscriminate use of cytotoxic drugs early in the course of the disease could inadvertently tip the balance against the host.

SELECTED READING

Levy JA: Human immunodeficiency viruses and the pathogenesis of AIDS. JAMA 261:2997, 1989

Evans LA, Levy JA: Characteristics of HIV infection and pathogenesis. Biochim Biophys Acta 989:237, 1989

Rosenberg ZF, Fauci AS: The immunopathogenesis of HIV infection. Adv Immunol 47:377, 1989

Fauci AS: The human immunodeficiency virus: Infectivity and mechanisms of pathogenesis. Science 239:617, 1988

Price RW et al: The brain in AIDS: Central nervous system HIV-1 infection and AIDS dementia complex. *Ibid:* 586

Clavel F: HIV-2, the West African AIDS virus. AIDS 1:135, 1987

Sattentau QJ: The role of the CD4 antigen in HIV infection and immune pathogenesis. AIDS 2(suppl):s11, 1988

Peterlin MB, Luciw PA: Molecular biology of HIV. *Ibid:* s29

Bolognesi DP: HIV antibodies and vaccine design. AIDS 3(suppl):s111, 1989

Levy JA (Ed): AIDS: Pathogenesis and Treatment. Marcel Dekker, New York, 1989

2 Immunopathogenesis of HIV Infection

PHILIP GREENBERG *University of Washington, Seattle*

Infectious exposure to HIV usually takes place through abrasion of a mucosal surface, such as the vaginal or rectal wall, or through intravenous inoculation during a transfusion, an IV drug injection, or a needle-stick injury. After this introduction into the host, the virus can take any of three paths. It may enter the circulation and remain there until it contacts and binds to a target cell expressing the CD4 molecule; it may adhere to CD4-expressing macrophages, Langerhans cells, or other types of cells and be transported extracellularly along with uninfected cells to regional lymph nodes; or it may directly infect a CD4+ cell and be transported to lymph nodes as an integral part of the infected cell. Presentation of viral antigens to lymphocytes in the lymph node eventuates in an immune response, culminating with the generation of CD4+ helper and effector cells, B cells secreting antibodies to HIV antigens, and CD8+ cytotoxic T cells capable of killing virally infected cells.

Up to this point, the natural history of HIV does not differ markedly from that of other lymphotropic pathogens. However, the HIV lentivirus has a number of unique features that not only permit escape from the host immune response but eventually lead to dysfunction and destruction of the immune system.

One feature facilitating this process is viral heterogeneity. Reverse transcriptase, the viral enzyme responsible for converting viral RNA into the DNA necessary for replication of the viral genome in an infected cell and the formation of new virions, is highly prone to error. Indeed, at the predicted error rate of approximately one out of every 10^4 base pairs, each progeny virus would be expected to differ genetically from its parent. Each of the consequent amino acid changes may be modest in itself, but as viral replication proceeds, an increasingly heterogeneous population of viruses evolves. Thus, the inoculum presented to a host upon initial exposure probably reflects a complex mixture of viral strains, which can differ in many properties such as cell tropism, replication efficiency, and cytopathology.

Let us examine, in a hypothetical scenario, the natural consequences of such replication heterogeneity. When an immunocompetent person—we shall call him A—receives an inoculum of HIV, the viral strains expressing highly immunogenic epitopes induce a protective host immune response. The resulting humoral and cellular immunity reduces the number of virions of these strains, but less immunogenic variants survive to produce progeny with a similar capacity to evade immunologic elimination. Within the next three years, A (who continues to be asymptomatic) passes the virus on to persons B and C. However, the proportion of less immunogenic, resistant HIV strains has risen markedly from the inoculum originally presented to A. Over the next year, B and C transmit HIV to new sexual partners D, E, and F. By the time these persons are infected, strains with reduced immunogenicity predominate, resulting in passage of potentially increasingly pathogenic viruses into the population.

Because no two human immune systems are exactly alike, a viral strain poorly immunogenic in one person may be immunogenic in others. Moreover, many other biologic factors contribute to the potential lethality of a virus. Nevertheless, experimental evidence is consistent with selection of increasingly pathogenic viruses at the individual and population level.

In the first place, it is widely recognized that HIV strains obtained from end-stage patients tend to be considerably more virulent than viruses obtained earlier in the clinical course. Second, viruses obtained from individuals with progressive disease often lack the immunogenic epitopes recognized by antibodies and CD8+ cytolytic T cells present during the asymptomatic period. Finally, recent data suggest that in geographic areas where the pathogen has been present for many years (e.g., sub-Saharan Africa), the strains commonly transmitted tend to be more virulent than those in areas where HIV was recently introduced.

A second distinctive feature of the lentiviruses is their capacity to remain sequestered within host cells for long periods with only sporadic bursts of reactivation (Figure 1). During these latent intervals, the host cell no longer expresses viral proteins. Because this portion of the HIV is not recognized by the immune system, the hidden viral population will not be diminished even if the patient is mounting a potentially effective response.

Eventually, the viruses in latently infected cells are reactivated—often as a consequence of a chance encounter with antigen or exposure to cytokines—and infectious virions are produced and released. By that time (and even though the patient may still feel healthy), the magnitude of the immune response specific for these virions may no longer be fully effective. The inefficiency of the immune response will be further exaggerated if the host has become immunocompromised. As viral replication proceeds, new errors are made and additional variant strains are produced, with some of the viruses retreating into latency once again. Each time this process is repeated, the burden of latent HIV increases, and the proportion of antigenic variants grows ominously larger.

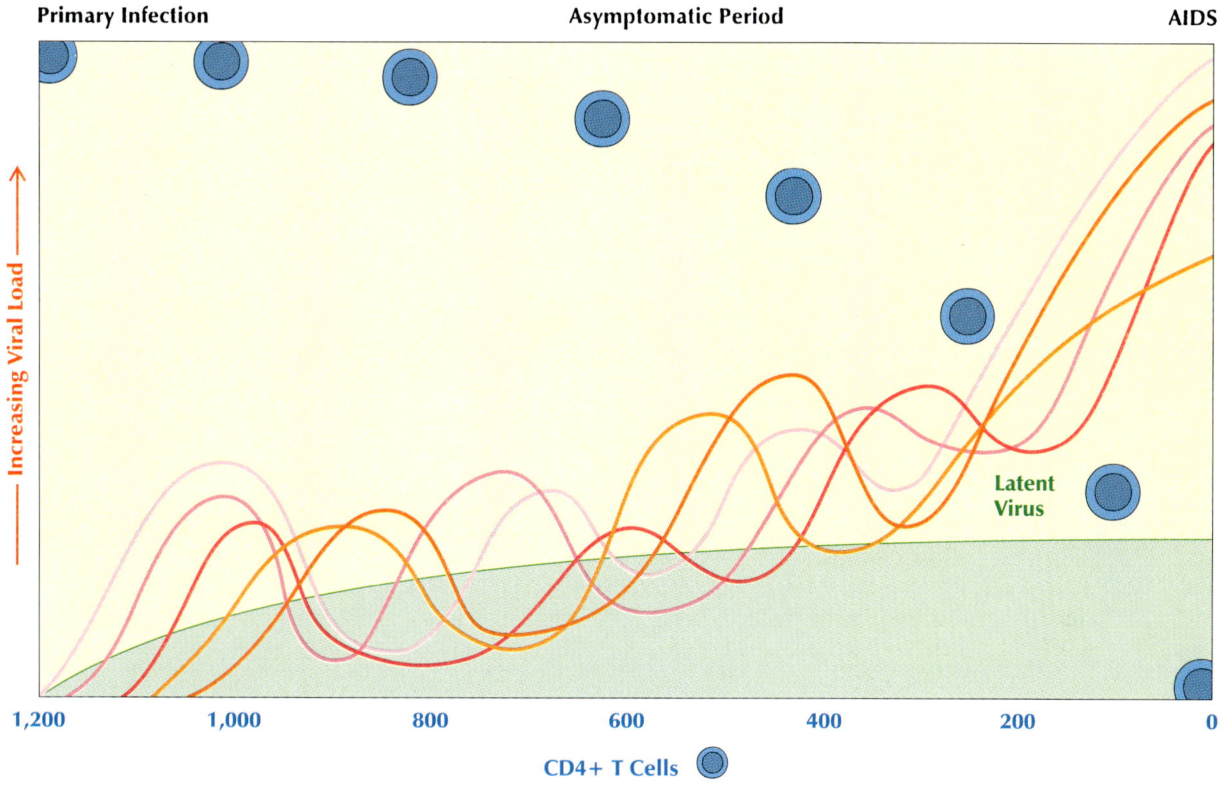

Figure 1 In the natural history of HIV infection, progression to AIDS is marked by a viral load that progressively increases in number and strain heterogeneity (symbolized by gradually rising curves). At the same time, the immune system steadily weakens, as reflected by a declining CD4 count. During primary infection, most of the virus is eliminated, but some persists—sequestered in latently infected cells or selected by immunologic resistance (reduced immunogenicity) during replication. Repeated episodes of viremia during the asymptomatic period result from reactivation of latent virus or outgrowth of resistant variants, or both. In time, mutations accumulate, so that the predominant strain will differ significantly from that of the initial inoculum. As the CD4 count continues to fall and the immune system becomes progressively less competent, the host is overwhelmed by resistant variants.

Effect on Hematopoietic Cells

The list of human cells susceptible to HIV encompasses a wide variety of cell types, including those of the brain, gastrointestinal tract, skin, and other organs. However, the largest reservoirs of latent virus are found in cells of hematopoietic lineage. When HIV has become established in bone marrow progenitor cells, such as monocyte precursors, promyelocytes, or possibly stem cells, every mature cell generated from the progenitor will be infected. Moreover, the functions of mature effector cells containing the HIV genome, such as CD4+ T cells and macrophages, will also be subverted by the expression of HIV genes. Thus, the cells that normally defend the organism from infection are rendered progressively less effective and ultimately become the major source of the infection (Figure 2).

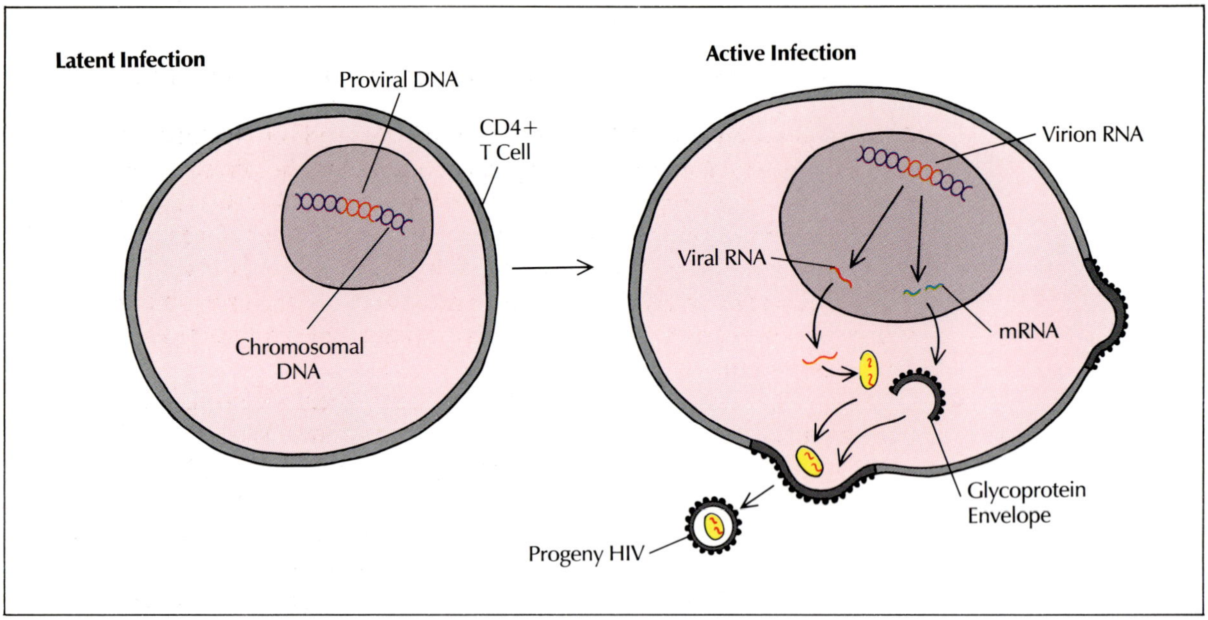

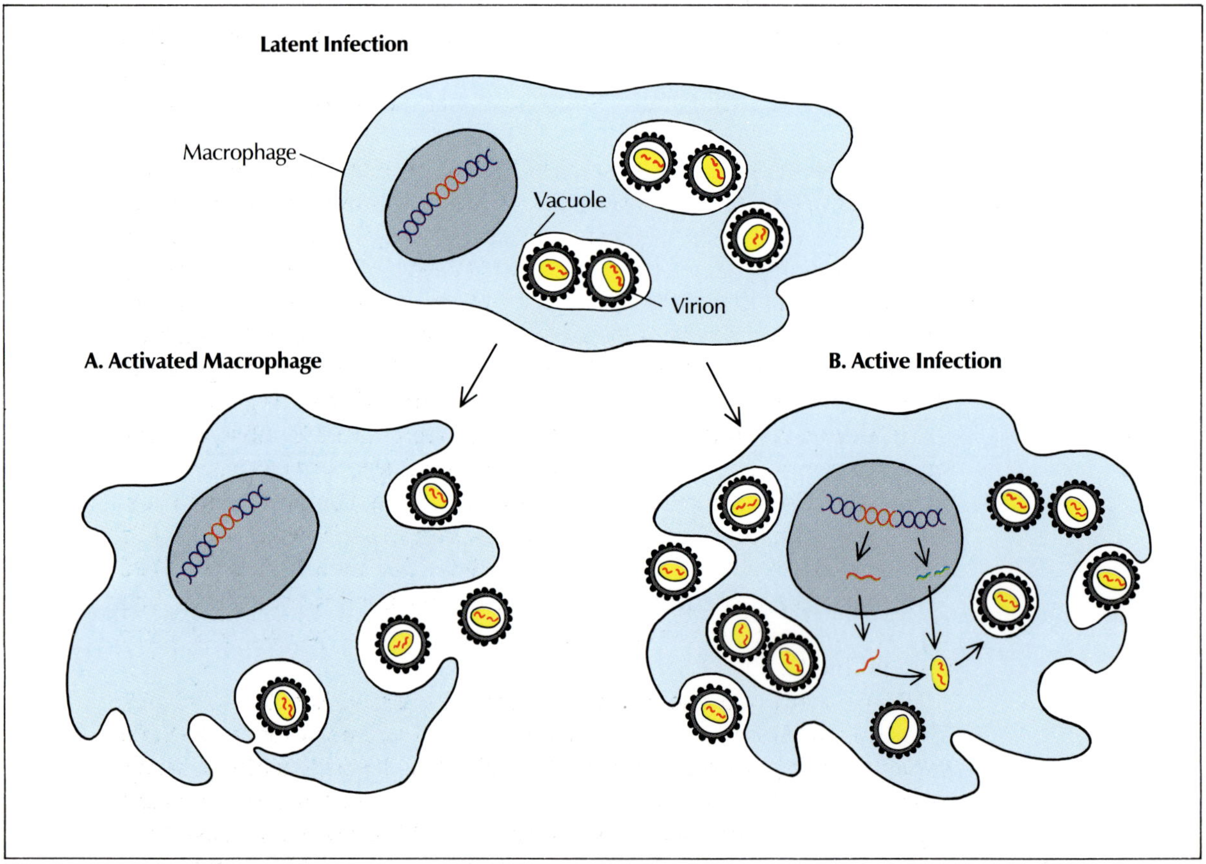

Figure 2 Among cell types susceptible to HIV infection, the CD4+ T cell (top) and the macrophage (bottom) are the most prominent targets. Each undergoes periods of latent and active infection with the virus. During latent infection of the CD4+ T cell, no viral genes are transcribed and translated, and no infectious virions are produced. All of these events occur during periods of active infection, and infectious viruses bud from the cell surface. In the latently infected macrophage, no viral genes are transcribed, but potentially infectious virions are sequestered within cytoplasmic vacuoles. On activation, infectious virions may be released from the vacuoles (A); alternatively, other activation events may prompt viral gene transcription and production of new virions for intravacuolar storage as well as virion release (B). Virions are not readily detected budding from the cell membrane of infected macrophages.

CD4+ T lymphocytes. HIV infection of cells depends on the binding of the virus's external envelope glycoprotein (gp120) to the lymphocyte-membrane-bound glycoprotein CD4, followed by internalization by the cell. CD4 is found in limited amounts on the surface of many cells but occurs in abundance on the helper/inducer subset of T cells. The resulting tropism of the virus for cells that regulate most host immune responses is in large part responsible for the devastating effects of HIV infection on the immune system.

Whenever the immune system of a seropositive patient is stimulated—whether by an opportunistic infection or by the common cold—CD4+ T cells are stimulated to produce the helper lymphokines necessary to promote an effective immune response. If, however, the activated CD4+ T cell contains latent virus, the viral genome will also be activated, and a period of viral production will follow. Additionally, the lymphokines produced by the stimulated T cells will activate macrophages, causing production and release of HIV from any macrophages infected by the virus. In sum, each normal immune response becomes an occasion for amplification of the HIV load, with resultant infection and elimination of previously normal CD4+ T cells and an incremental loss of their normal effector functions (Figure 3).

Potential mechanisms for CD4+ T-cell depletion are numerous. These include cell death due to accumulation of unintegrated HIV DNA; toxicity of a viral gene product such as gp120; syncytia formation and cell death following fusion of normal CD4+ cells with cells expressing gp120; lysis of infected cells due to membrane damage from viral budding; immunologic lysis of infected cells or of uninfected cells that have become coated with free gp120; autoimmunity, in which the response to the viral envelope protein gp160 recognizes a homologous region of class II molecules normally expressed on activated CD4+ T cells; autoimmune prevention of CD4+ T-cell proliferation due to immune responses to a region of interleukin-2 (the T-cell growth factor) homologous to portions of gp120; interference with the development of new CD4+ T cells from immature precursors owing to binding of autoantibodies or gp120 to class II molecules; destruction of early bone marrow precursors; and cell death resulting from a gp120-induced chronic partial activation state (Table 1).

While many of those mechanisms involve actual infection of CD4+ T cells, roughly half relate to disruptions in the maturation, functional capacity, or expansion of uninfected cells. The developmental progression of T cells from immature precursors to mature effector cells is a highly ordered sequence, and interference with these events results in cell death. Thus, if the CD4 molecules on a developing T cell are occupied because of bound gp120 at the critical point when interaction with class II molecules on thymic epithelial or stromal cells is essential, the result is likely to be rapid cell death. Alternatively, autoantibodies to IL-2 might interfere with the effective delivery of a growth signal at the necessary time. Even after CD4+ T cells have matured, the binding of gp120 to CD4 can result in delivery of an intracellular signal and chronic partial

Figure 3. Normal Effector Functions of the CD4+ T Cell

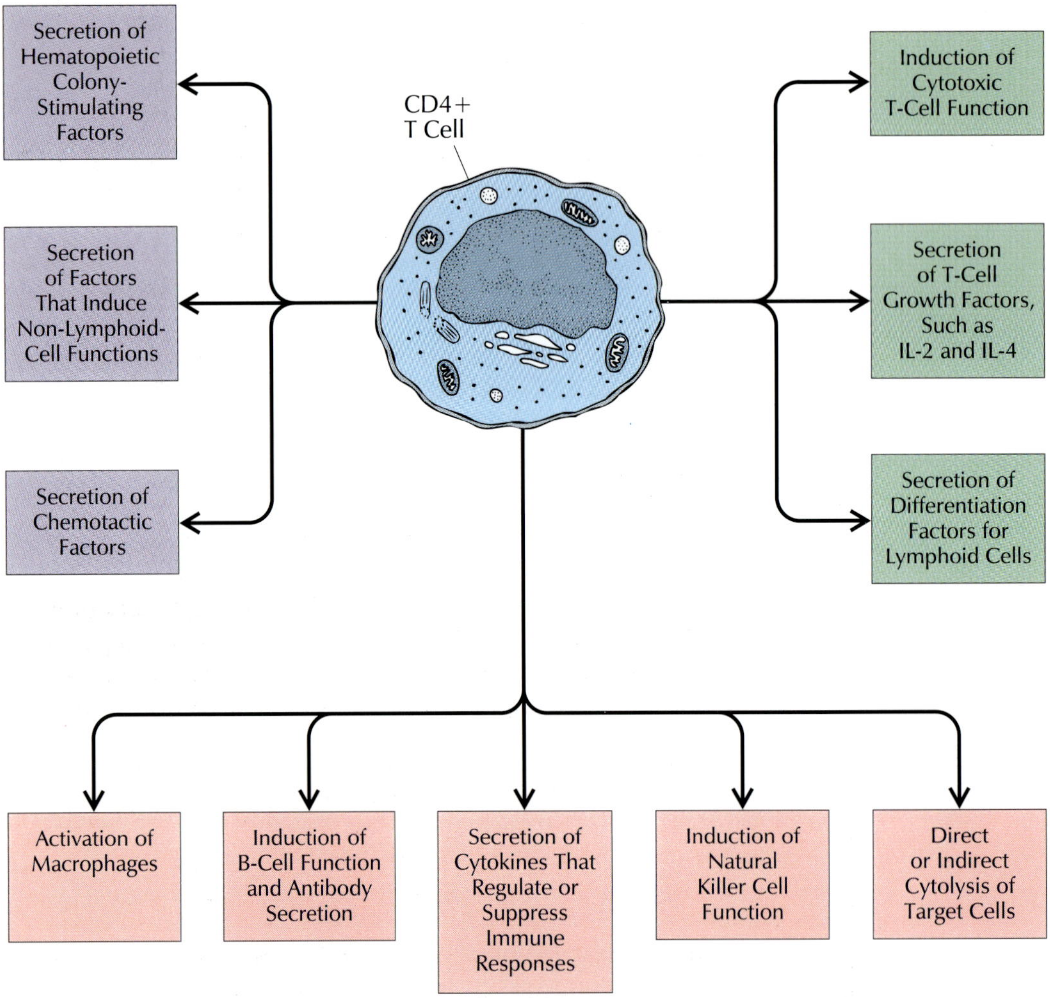

activation, leading to dysfunction and ultimately death of the abnormally activated cell. These problems, leading to gradual diminution of the number of mature CD4+ effector cells, are further compounded by lysis of early bone marrow precursors of CD4+ cells.

By the time a significant decline in the number of CD4+ T cells is noted, the HIV-seropositive patient has already experienced a consider-

Table 1. Potential Mechanisms for Depletion of CD4+ T Cells by HIV Infection

- Accumulation of unintegrated intracellular HIV DNA
- Expression of toxic HIV gene product (e.g., gp160)
- Syncytia formation (e.g., fusion of normal CD4+ T cells with infected cells expressing gp120)
- Lysis of infected CD4+ T cells by membrane damage from viral budding
- Lysis of infected CD4+ T cells by virus-specific immunologic mechanisms
- Immune-mediated lysis of normal CD4+ T cells coated with gp120
- Autoimmune response to region of class II molecule homologous to gp120 or gp41
- Autoimmune response to region of IL-2 (T-cell growth factor) homologous to gp120
- Interference with generation of new CD4+ T cells (e.g., by prevention of ontogeny due to binding of autoantibodies to class II molecules or binding of gp120 to CD4 molecules)
- Destruction of early bone marrow progenitor cells
- Dysfunction and death resulting from chronic partial CD4+ T-cell activation (gp120 binding to CD4)

able loss of CD4+ effector function (Table 2). This loss may be demonstrated by the blunted responses of CD4+ T cells from healthy-appearing HIV-infected patients to antigen stimuli. When tested in vitro, the cells show reduced clonal expansion, decreased production of lym-

Table 2. Functional Abnormalities of T Cells in HIV-Infected Hosts

In Vitro

- Decreased response to antigens, with reduced lymphokine production and proliferation
- Impaired triggering of both CD4+ and CD8+ T-cell effector functions
- Reduced expression of IL-2 receptor following stimulation (with associated reduction in response to IL-2)
- Elevated spontaneous proliferation
- Reduced ability of individual cells to expand clonally following stimulation
- Poor helper function for B-cell responses
- Decreased virus-specific cytotoxic responses

In Vivo Responses

- Partial activation of CD4+ and CD8+ T cells
- Preferential loss of CD4+ T cells of memory phenotype
- Decreased delayed hypersensitivity responses
- Increased susceptibility to opportunistic infections

phokines such as IL-2, poor assistance to B cells (as evidenced by inadequate specific antibody production), and diminished delayed-type hypersensitivity reactions.

The blunting of the immune function of CD4+ T cells is particularly evident in the mature memory CD4+ T-cell subset—the population that ordinarily generates rapid, effective responses to antigenic stimuli to which it has been previously exposed. In healthy patients, such responses predominate over those of naive T cells reacting to antigen for the first time. However, because HIV preferentially infects activated T cells and integration of the viral genome occurs predominantly in cells replicating endogenous DNA, cells that have previously responded to antigen are more likely than naive cells to be infected or to have been depleted. Additionally, the initial immune response of CD4+ T cells requires presentation of antigen by cells such as macrophages, which may themselves be infected and will pass the infection to the responding T cell. Thus, HIV-seropositive persons tend to have a proportionately greater incidence of relatively immature, unprimed cells and correspondingly deficient memory responses.

CD8+ T lymphocytes. Disturbances of CD8+ cytotoxic T-cell responses, like those of CD4+ T cells, become apparent early in the course of HIV infection. The disturbances include reduced clonal expansion following activation, decreased response following normal trigger signals, and chronic partial activation. During the initial phase of lymphadenopathy, the CD8+ population may appear to rise, owing to temporarily increased activation in the lymph nodes and release of cytotoxic T cells into the peripheral blood. However, patients with full-blown AIDS generally demonstrate a loss of CD8+ cells, albeit on a much smaller scale than the loss of CD4+ helper cells, which are the actual targets of the virus.

In patients who are asymptomatic or just beginning to be symptomatic, part of the blunted cytotoxic T-cell response detected in vitro may be corrected by the addition of exogenous IL-2, which compensates for inadequate production of this growth factor by a deficient CD4+ T-cell response. However, as the disease progresses, supplemental IL-2 cannot fully compensate for the decline in CD4+ helper functions. Presumably, this change reflects chronic dysfunction of the CD8+ subset due to aberrant activation.

With advancing disease, opportunities for concurrent contact with mature, fully functional helper CD4+ cells during the activation of CD8+ T cells by recognition of antigen become increasingly limited. Thus, CD8+ T cells will frequently not receive all the signals necessary for activation of effector functions. As a result, CD8-mediated responses in general and HIV-specific cytotoxicity in particular diminish dramatically. In patients with late-stage AIDS, virus-specific cytotoxicity is often impossible to detect, despite the presence of a numerically large CD8+ cell population.

Macrophages. Although CD4 molecules are expressed in smaller quantities on macrophages than on CD4+ T lymphocytes, macrophages still constitute an important reservoir of HIV in infected patients. Indeed, latently infected macrophages containing huge numbers of virions packaged into vesicles can often be identified, and activation of these macrophages can result in release of infectious virus. Analysis of different HIV isolates suggests that certain viral strains are extremely monocytotropic, whereas others appear to infect macrophages only uncommonly. Gene-shuffling experiments suggest that these differences in target specificity reflect acquired genetic changes in the virus, with resultant changes in the gp120 molecule.

Significant functional abnormalities may be seen in uninfected as well as infected macrophages from HIV-seropositive persons. Among the abnormalities found in vitro are diminished reactivity to triggering stimuli, with consequent impaired secretion of monokines and defective antigen presentation to T cells; partial activation, with inappropriate "leaking" (spontaneous secretion) of small quantities of IL-1, IL-6, tumor necrosis factor, and other monokines; diminished chemotaxis and phagocytosis; inadequate production of IL-1 in response to appropriate stimuli such as phagocytosis of antigen; decreased expression of MHC class II surface antigens (which provide the necessary context for antigen recognition by CD4+ T cells); and reduced reticuloendothelial clearance (Table 3).

The virus also inhibits macrophage effector functions responsible for resistance to infectious agents. The diminished intracellular and extracellular killing activities of macrophages encourage the growth of fungi and parasites such as *Candida albicans*, *Toxoplasma gondii*, and *Giardia lamblia*.

B lymphocytes. Abnormalities of B-cell function are also apparent early in the course of HIV infection. Although the majority of these disturbances are clearly related to disruptions of T-cell signaling, some appear to reflect a direct influence of the virus on B cells themselves. Infect-

Table 3. Functional Abnormalities of Macrophages in HIV-Infected Hosts

Elevated spontaneous secretion of IL-1, PGE_2, TNFα, and IL-6 (may reflect stimulation by gp120)

Poor response to stimuli (i.e., decreased production of IL-1 following stimulation)

Impaired chemotaxis and phagocytosis

Defective intra- and extracellular killing of pathogens

Decreased expression of class II antigens—poor induction of class II expression in response to γ-interferon

Diminished capacity to present antigen to T cells

ed persons demonstrate polyclonal activation of B cells, as reflected in vitro by increased spontaneous proliferation and immunoglobulin synthesis and in vivo by chronically elevated serum immunoglobulin levels.

Yet despite this frenetic activity, the actual responsiveness of B cells to specific antigenic stimuli is sharply curtailed. In vitro proliferative responses to stimulation with antigen and mitogen are generally poor, and immunoglobulin synthesis following stimulation with pokeweed mitogen is decreased. In vivo, these functional abnormalities are reflected by inadequate antibody responses to infection or immunization with antigens such as pneumococcal polysaccharides and by poor isotype switching from primary IgM responses to secondary IgG responses. Abnormal regulation of B-cell function is also evident, as reflected by the presence of circulating immature B cells, immune complexes, and autoantibodies (Table 4).

The question of why B lymphocytes are persistently activated in patients infected by HIV has puzzled investigators for some time. Potentially, the chronic leakage of small quantities of macrophage products such as IL-1 and IL-6 as well as the abnormal production of stimulatory and regulatory cytokines by CD4+ T cells could result in chronic low-level activation of B lymphocytes. Then too, TAT, a viral regulatory protein that induces HIV gene activation, is also capable of activating lymphoid cells, and uptake of this protein from extracellular fluid might provide a signal for the nonspecific activation of B cells. Whatever the relative importance of these factors, the end result is that infected patients experience disruptions of humoral immunity.

Table 4. Functional Abnormalities of B Cells in HIV-Infected Hosts

In Vitro

- Increased spontaneous polyclonal Ig synthesis without stimulation
- Increased proliferation in response to B-cell growth factors
- Reduced reactivity to B-cell mitogens (T-cell dependent or independent)
- Impaired response to new antigens
- Impaired response by memory B cells to antigens
- Decreased responsiveness to regulatory signals

In Vivo

- Poor antibody response to infection or immunization
- Poor isotype switching
- Elevated serum Ig (polyclonal) levels
- Presence of immature B cells in periphery
- Presence of circulating immune complexes
- Presence of autoantibodies

The persistent activation of B lymphocytes almost certainly contributes to the high incidence of B-cell malignancies seen in patients with AIDS. Approximately 50% of these lymphomas contain Epstein-Barr virus genomes—a finding consistent with the increased risk of immortalizing infection in proliferating B cells, and consistent, too, with an inadequate host T-cell response to viruses such as Epstein-Barr virus.

Natural killer cells. To an immunocompromised patient unable to summon an adequate defensive response by T and B lymphocytes, a potent natural killer cell response would clearly be of great benefit. Unfortunately, in the case of HIV even this rudimentary form of resistance is suboptimal. To be sure, neither the overall number of NK cells nor the ability of these effector cells to bind to targets appears to be diminished. Nevertheless, HIV-seropositive patients show a definite decrease in NK cytolytic activity, with reduced cytotoxicity per effector cell and impaired lysis of tumor cell lines and virally infected cells.

The problem seems to reflect compromised function of cytolytic mechanisms, such as that effecting release of NK cytolytic factor. Under normal circumstances, a reorientation of the microtubular system of the NK cell takes place shortly after binding to the target cell, resulting in polarization of intracellular structures for delivery of the cytolytic signal at the site of contact between the NK cell and its target. In HIV-infected persons, this cytoskeletal rearrangement fails to occur.

Because mature NK cells are not infectible with HIV (although their precursors may be) and do not typically express CD4, there has been considerable speculation over the mechanism by which the abnormality in microtubular rearrangement develops. One suggestion is that diminished production of IL-2 and γ-interferon by infected CD4+ helper T cells produces a chronic dysfunction of the NK cell population. Another proposed mechanism involves aberrant, partial activation through stimulation of two receptors expressed by the majority of NK cells. The first is a receptor for the Fc region of immunoglobulin, which may bind the circulating immune complexes found in HIV-seropositive patients and produce partial activation of NK cells at times when an appropriate target cell is nowhere in sight. The second is the receptor for the hormone known as vasoactive intestinal peptide (VIP), which may, after binding its ligand, dampen NK cytolytic activity through elevation of intracellular cyclic AMP levels. (Whether VIP is the natural ligand for this receptor or merely is homologous to the true ligand remains unclear. However, VIP does have homology with a portion of the gp120 molecule, and it is suspected that gp120 can also bind to the receptor and decrease lytic activity by direct activation.)

An Underlying Mechanism?

The global nature of the immunologic dysfunction seen in HIV infection has led investigators to hypothesize that failure of a single, basic biologic mechanism may underlie many of the changes previously described. Lymphocytes communicate with each other either by direct cell-cell interaction or by secretion of cytokines, and they respond to such messages, delivered at the cell membrane, by the transduction of signals to the inside of the cell. The generation of most effector responses requires the orderly delivery and processing of multiple signals, and alterations in this process can lead to a dysfunctional response.

Studies analyzing the signal pathways in the lymphoid cells of HIV-seropositive patients have suggested that abnormalities begin to appear very early in the disease. Some of these investigations have involved measurements of the turnover of inositol triphosphate and inositol tetraphosphate, which function as second messengers in cells through the regulation of intracellular calcium levels. (The messengers promote release of calcium from microsomal stores or entry of calcium into the cell through the plasma membrane.) Other studies have measured intracellular calcium directly.

The results indicate that many cells infected by HIV are not in a truly resting phase: They show chronically elevated levels of intracellular calcium. One major consequence of a persistent elevation would be a failure to respond to normal triggering stimuli, such as receptor binding, with an appropriate increase in calcium. Remarkably, chronic elevations of intracellular calcium are found not only in HIV-infected hematopoietic and neural cells but also in uninfected cells from HIV-seropositive patients.

This phenomenon may well reflect any of a number of abnormal signaling events, such as binding of gp120 to CD4 on the cell, which (through linkage to a G protein or to an intracellular tyrosine kinase) delivers an intracellular signal. Alternatively, uptake of virally produced proteins, such as TAT, might result in activation by inducing transcription of cellular genes. The result is likely to be interruption of the orderly cellular activation process and premature, partial activation. The failure of these partially activated cells to receive the subsequent signals necessary for expression of an effector response could result in cells that do not respond normally when they encounter an appropriate stimulus. It could also cause the cells to become increasingly dysfunctional and die.

Implications for Drug Therapy

We have described how exposure to HIV produces a wide range of functional abnormalities in immunohematopoietic cells—even when the cells themselves do not actually become infected. Moreover, by residing in cells involved in immune responses, the infection gains the ability to amplify and progress as the host responds to normal environmental stimuli and pathogens. With each exposure of infected cells to a stimulating antigen, additional free viral particles are released, new variants are produced, and stores of latent HIV are increased. The proportion of mature effector cells free of the virus gradually diminishes, along with the availability of new helper/inducer CD4+ T cells essential in augmenting and regulating most immune responses. In these ways, the immune system becomes increasingly dysfunctional, setting the stage for opportunistic infections. At the same time, the diminished efficacy of the immune response prolongs the duration of each infective episode. The resulting extension of specific and nonspecific stimulation of the immune system provides heightened opportunity for the virus to proliferate and spread to previously uninfected cells.

Effective therapy thus requires prevention of viral replication and abrogation of the expression of viral gene products. Treatment of the patient with an antiretroviral agent such as zidovudine, may substantially diminish the viral burden and prolong the asymptomatic period. However, the great variance of HIV strains and the resistance of latently infected cells to drug therapy mean that the effectiveness of zidovudine tends to decline after two or three years. More powerful antiretrovirals and drugs targeted at different stages in the retroviral life cycle should help in delaying progression to AIDS, but actual cure will not be possible until a way is found of eliminating the stored virus. Ideally, this might be accomplished early in the disease—when the viral burden is small and immunity is relatively intact—by treating patients both with drugs such as cytokines that can stimulate viral gene expression in latently infected cells and with more classic therapy involving agents that kill infected cells and prevent viral replication or integration.

SELECTED READING

Rosenberg ZF, Fauci AS: The immunopathogenesis of HIV infection. Adv Immunol 47:377, 1989

McCune JM: HIV-1: The infective process in vivo. Cell 64:351, 1991

Pinching AJ, Nye KE: Defective signal transduction: A common pathway for cellular dysfunction in HIV infection? Immunol Today 11:256, 1990

McChesney MB, Oldstone MBA: Virus-induced immunosuppression: Infections with measles virus and human immunodeficiency virus. Adv Immunol 45:335, 1989

Walker BD, Plata F: Cytotoxic T lymphocytes against HIV. AIDS 4:177, 1990

Meltzer MS et al: Macrophages and the human immunodeficiency virus. Immunol Today 11:217, 1990

Phillips RE et al: Human immunodeficiency virus genetic variation that can escape cytotoxic T cell recognition. Nature 354:453, 1991

Habeshaw JA et al: AIDS pathogenesis: HIV envelope and its interaction with cell proteins. Immunol Today 11:418, 1990

3 The Changing Epidemiology of HIV Transmission

KING K. HOLMES *University of Washington, Seattle*

As of April 1991, more than 345,000 cases of AIDS had been reported to the World Health Organization. Because of chronic underreporting in developing countries, however, the true count probably exceeds 1 million cases in adults. In addition, it is estimated that by early 1991, more than 500,000 pediatric AIDS cases may have occurred, resulting from perinatal transmission. WHO estimates that at least 8 to 10 million adults had been infected with the human immunodeficiency virus by early 1991, and another million children had been infected. Whereas an overwhelming percentage of these infections were sexually acquired—the majority, perhaps 60%, through heterosexual contact and 15% homosexually—an additional 10% were acquired perinatally. Globally, heterosexual transmissions are outnumbering all other categories and may account for more than 80% of HIV transmissions by the end of the decade. At the same time, we anticipate a gradual flattening of the transmission curves for homosexual men and intravenous drug users, as well as a continued decline in the number of new HIV infections attributable to contaminated blood products. Nonetheless, WHO projects that with rapid spread of the epidemic in southern and southeastern Asia, the cumulative total number of HIV-infected adults will reach 30 million by the year 2000, with an additional 10 million pediatric cases.

The rising infection rate among women and children is particularly worrisome (Table 1). A recent survey by James Chin of the WHO Global Program on AIDS concluded that the HIV pandemic will kill 3 million or more women and children during the 1990s. In New York City, as in many urban population centers of sub-Saharan Africa, AIDS has become the leading cause of death in women aged 20 to 40. High rates of

Table 1. Estimated HIV Infection Rate Among 15- to 49-Year-Old Women

Region	*Prevalence (Per 100,000 Women)*	*Estimated Number of Cases*
Sub-Saharan Africa	2,500	> 2,500,000
South America	200	200,000
North America	140	100,000
Western Europe	70	60,000
Australia and New Zealand	70	< 4,000
South Asia	30	200,000
North Africa	20	< 10,000
Eastern Europe	< 5	< 4,000

Adapted from Chin J, 1990

rapidly progressive pediatric HIV infection have already reversed much of the progress that has been made over the past 20 years in reducing infant and child mortality in some developing countries. During the 1990s, child mortality rates in some sub-Saharan African countries are expected to increase by up to 50%. (Infected children progress to AIDS more rapidly than infected adults, although not as rapidly as once thought.) In addition to the 10 million children who will be infected with HIV by the year 2000, another 10 million uninfected children will be orphaned.

Four Global Patterns

Four distinct patterns of HIV transmission have been described by WHO (Table 2). Although useful conceptually, they provide only a broad brushstroke outline of the current status of the epidemic in a particular geographic region and do not necessarily represent the future of the epidemic in that region. Furthermore, HIV infection occurs disproportionately in certain high-risk groups. Hence, seroprevalence may differ markedly between neighboring countries, urban and rural areas within a single country, or social strata within an urban population.

Table 2. Global Patterns of HIV-1 Infection

Pattern I: Predominantly homosexual men and intravenous drug users (IVDUs); gradual increase of heterosexual and perinatal transmission—e.g., North America, Western Europe, Australia, and New Zealand

Pattern II: Predominantly non-IVDU heterosexuals; female-male ratio approaches or surpasses 1:1; perinatal transmission a major problem—e.g., sub-Saharan Africa, parts of the Caribbean, and parts of Asia

Pattern I/II: Currently evolving from predominantly homosexual and bisexual to heterosexual transmission—e.g., Brazil, Honduras, and Chile

Pattern III: HIV infection still relatively uncommon; infected homosexual men, prostitutes, and IVDUs are a rapidly growing problem in some areas—e.g., Eastern Europe, North Africa, Middle East, parts of Asia, and the Pacific (excluding Australia and New Zealand)

Pattern I encompasses the industrialized nations of North America and Western Europe, as well as Australia and New Zealand. In these areas, between 80% and 90% of HIV transmission has been attributable to male homosexual contact or intravenous drug use (IVDU). The female-male ratio of reported AIDS cases has remained about 1:10 to 1:15, and pediatric AIDS cases have been relatively fewer in number than in other parts of the world. This pattern is beginning to change, however, as heterosexual transmission of HIV increases and the number of new cases among homosexual men declines.

In pattern II areas of sub-Saharan Africa, viral transmission has been predominantly heterosexual since the epidemic began, which was probably in the mid- to late 1970s. The female-male ratio of reported AIDS cases is about 1:1, and perinatal transmission is already a devastating problem. High rates of heterosexually transmitted HIV have also been reported throughout the Caribbean (especially in Haiti and the Bahamas).

Although homosexual and bisexual contact remains the major route of HIV transmission in Latin America, the picture in many countries (e.g., Honduras, Brazil, Chile) is gradually changing with increasing heterosexual spread of the virus. As a result, such countries have been reclassified as pattern I/II.

Finally, in the so-called pattern III areas of Eastern Europe, North Africa, the Middle East, the Pacific (excluding Australia and New Zealand), and parts of Asia, HIV is a relatively recent arrival, and viral prevalence remains low. However, rapid spread of infection is now being documented among intravenous drug users and homosexual men in southeastern Asia, and heterosexual transmission is increasing rapidly in Thailand and India, where high rates of infection have been found in female prostitutes.

The patterns outlined above refer to distribution of the more common form of the human immunodeficiency virus, HIV-1. HIV-2 has become endemic in the West African nations of Senegal, Guinea-Bissau, Mali, Burkina Faso, and Ivory Coast, as well as Angola and Mozambique. High prevalence rates in female prostitutes and STD clinic populations in these countries suggest that like HIV-1, HIV-2 is spread primarily through heterosexual transmission. However, the rate at which HIV-2 infection progresses to AIDS may be somewhat slower than that of HIV-1. Although introduced into West Africa more recently than HIV-2, HIV-1 appears to be spreading more rapidly via sexual transmission, and West Africans infected with HIV-1 tend to be younger than those infected with HIV-2. Although isolated cases of HIV-2 infection have been identified in other African nations as well as in Europe, Brazil, and North America, most affected persons have either lived among or shared intravenous needles with West Africans.

Varying Transmission Dynamics

Obviously, the transmission dynamics of HIV vary considerably from population to population. Efforts to understand why the virus has gained a firm foothold among homosexual men in industrialized countries and heterosexual men and (especially) women in some developing countries, but not in others, have led to identification of a number of factors that appear to promote HIV spread: longer duration of the epidemic; receptive anorectal or (to a lesser extent) vaginal intercourse; numerous sexual partners or high-risk partners; prostitution; IV drug use; sex exchanged for crack cocaine; presence of other sexually transmitted diseases; absence of circumcision; and receipt of contaminated blood products.

The importance of sexual activity as a factor in the rapid spread of the virus among homosexual and bisexual men in the United States and other Western countries is well known. Although homosexual practices are generally taboo in sub-Saharan Africa, heterosexual intercourse with multiple partners and female prostitution are extremely common. In one study of prostitutes in a slum area of Nairobi, Francis Plummer and co-workers found that the prevalence of HIV infection rose from 4% to more than 85% in less than five years.

Estimates of the efficiency of HIV transmission have ranged widely in different populations. In the United States and other pattern I areas, the probability of transmission per partner contact appears to be considerably higher among homosexual men than among heterosexuals—a difference that may largely reflect the high transmission efficiency of receptive anorectal intercourse.

Early studies of monogamous heterosexual couples in which one partner had acquired HIV infection through clotting factor concentrate or blood transfusion found that female-to-male or male-to-female transmission was less than 20%, even after several years of exposure. More recent reports suggest that with still longer exposure, approximately 50% to 60% of heterosexual partners ultimately seroconvert. The risk of male-to-female transmission appears to be somewhat greater than the converse.

Risk of transmission also appears to rise as the index patient becomes progressively immunosuppressed and plasma concentrations of virus increase. A low peripheral blood CD4 lymphocyte count is therefore probably a strong predictor of increased efficiency of sexual transmission, regardless of sexual practices. In one study from Kinshasa, Zaire, the rate of perinatal transmission, ascertained after two years of follow-up, also correlated universally with the CD4 lymphocyte count in the mother. It is theorized that the high transmission efficiency of HIV among heterosexuals in central Africa may be partly a function of the relatively long duration of the epidemic and the high proportion of infected persons with advanced immunosuppression.

The role of other STDs as cofactors in the transmission of HIV has been well documented in Africa and is becoming increasingly apparent in the Americas. Genital or anorectal ulcers (chancroid, syphilis, herpes, and granuloma inguinale) have been associated with increased risk of sexual transmission of HIV, presumably because they provide convenient portals through which the virus may be shed or inoculated. Mononuclear cells at the base of the ulcer are thought to be especially susceptible to infection by HIV. Endocervical infections by *Chlamydia trachomatis* or *Neisseria gonorrhoeae* have similarly been implicated as facilitating sexual transmission of HIV, perhaps by causing cervical inflammation and micro-ulceration.

Regarding the three major vaginal infections of adults—trichomoniasis, candidiasis, and bacterial vaginosis—only trichomoniasis has been correlated with an increased risk of HIV infection. However, the lactobacillus hydrogen peroxide–halide-peroxidase vaginal microbicidal system has recently been shown to be active against HIV, and the lactobacilli that colonize the vagina in bacterial vaginosis lack this microbicidal system.

Recent evidence in humans and lower primates indicates that dendritic cells in vaginal epithelium are particularly susceptible to HIV infection. The reasons for this require further study. Possible factors include the influence of other vaginal infections, use of spermicides, frequency of intercourse, and normal developmental changes. Finally, it has been shown that HIV is shed from genital ulcers. The effects of cervicitis, urethritis, and vaginitis on genital shedding of HIV also require further study.

A number of investigators have reported a negative association between the practice of circumcision among the various ethnic groups throughout Africa and the distribution of HIV. In a prospective study of Kenyan men who presented at an STD clinic after prostitute contact, subjects not circumcised had an eightfold higher risk of HIV seroconversion than did circumcised subjects. There was also a positive correlation between absence of circumcision and rates of chancroid and other genital ulcer diseases that increase the risk of acquiring HIV. The apparent effect of circumcision in reducing HIV risk may well be at least partly indirect. However, the studies in Kenya found that absence of circumcision was associated with HIV infection independent of genital ulcers, indicating both direct and indirect relations with HIV.

Although sexual contact is certainly the most common mode of HIV transmission, parenteral exposure to contaminated blood or blood products is a continuing problem, especially in developing countries. Retrospective studies of persons who received blood before 1985, when HIV screening was instituted in the United States, showed that receiving a contaminated unit of blood was associated with a 90% or greater probability of infection. Transmission from contaminated intravenous needles is considerably less efficient, presumably because much smaller inocula of blood are involved.

Although no blood screening system is foolproof (potential donors may still test negative for HIV antibody for several weeks after infection), the current U.S. blood supply is now considered to be very safe. In contrast, seroprevalence rates among blood donors in some AIDS-endemic areas of Africa remain as high as 15% to 18%, as screening of donors for HIV is not yet universal. In some areas of Asia, even where the overall prevalence of HIV infection in the general population remains low, up to 10% of paid blood donors have been found to be seropositive. Efforts to replace paid donors with volunteer donors are proceeding as blood screening for HIV is being introduced.

African women and children have been found to be at particular risk of parenteral infection because blood is frequently administered during pregnancy and childbirth, as well as later to counter pediatric anemia associated with nutritional deficiencies, hemoglobinopathies, and infections such as malaria.

In studying the association between malaria, blood transfusion, and HIV seropositivity in a pediatric population in a hospital in Kinshasa, Zaire, A. E. Greenberg and colleagues found that, in the course of a year, 561 children admitted with malaria received HIV-positive blood transfusions. More recently, the blood-safety picture in the African AIDS belt has improved, and HIV antibody screening programs are now in place in most large population centers.

Isolated outbreaks of nosocomially transmitted HIV have also been documented in the Soviet Union and Romania, where they have been linked with reuse of contaminated needles and syringes and (in Romania) transfusion of unscreened blood.

It is clear that the potential for similar nosocomial transmission of HIV by contaminated reusable equipment or contaminated blood products exists throughout Africa, Asia, and Latin America, where disposable equipment is lacking and infection control policies and blood banking practices are often not optimal. However, nosocomial transmission is difficult to detect in these regions.

This is creating a major dilemma in public health. On the one hand, it is clear that the vast majority of infections are transmitted sexually or by IVDU and that only prevention of these modes of transmission will have a real impact on the epidemic. On the other hand, the public tends to demand that blood and blood products (and even health personnel) be free of HIV, and the medical profession, politicians, and donor agencies find it easier and less controversial to clean up the blood supply and deal with nosocomial infection control practices (both are undeniably important) than to confront the greater problems of sexual and IVDU transmission.

Regional Trends for the 1990s

Europe. Between March 1989 and March 1990, the cumulative number of AIDS cases reported to WHO by the 32 countries of the European region increased by 61.9%. This continued the trend established in the early 1980s (Figure 1). The largest relative increases came from Eastern Europe (Romania, 4,680%; Poland, 338%; USSR, 271%; Bulgaria, 133%), where few AIDS cases had been reported previously. Clearly, improved surveillance was one factor in the change. Another, at least in Romania and the USSR, was increased nosocomial transmission of HIV.

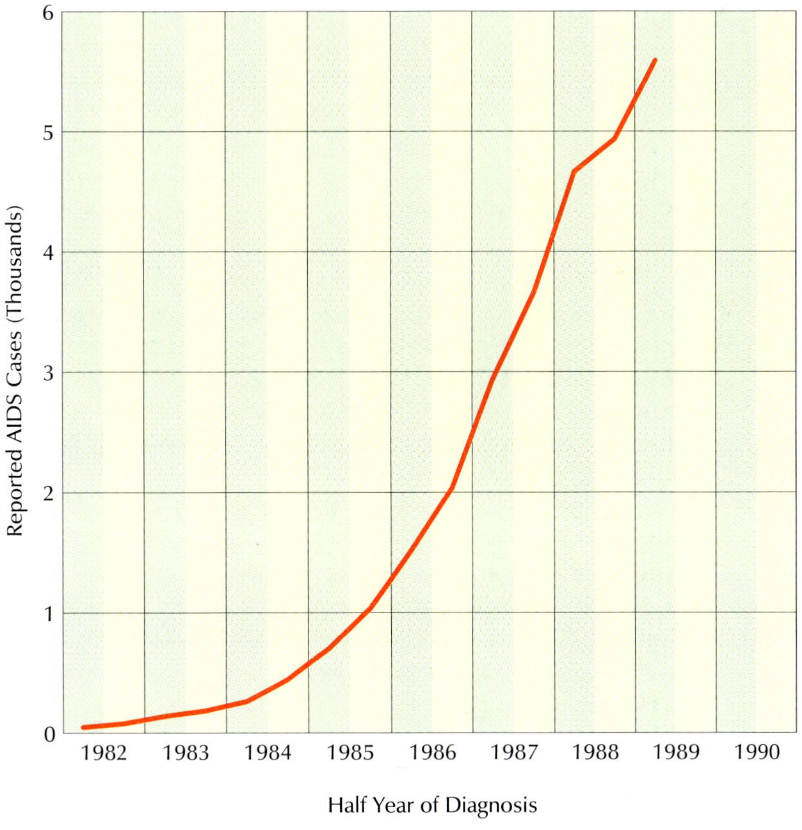

Figure 1 The number of AIDS cases reported in Europe has steadily risen since 1982, as shown by WHO data collected by half year of diagnosis (reports as of March 1990 were incomplete for the second half of 1989 and the first half of 1990).

In the USSR, prior to the 1991 coup attempt, concern had also been expressed that the nation's vast network of educational, economic, and military assistance programs could become a pipeline for HIV transmission. Sexual contact with HIV-infected persons from pattern II areas has been associated with a high percentage of Soviet AIDS cases; although the absolute numbers are not large, they bear watching. Similarly, rates of indigenous homosexual and IVDU transmission appear to have been very low in most Eastern European countries prior to the 1989–1990 breakdown of the Iron Curtain, but the potential for more rapid spread has increased with the opening of borders to the West. Exceptions have included Poland, which has seen a growing HIV problem among heroin users, particularly in Warsaw, and Hungary, where a number of cases of AIDS had already been seen in homosexual men by 1990. It is now hoped that the USSR and the Eastern European countries, like other pattern III countries, will be able to benefit from lessons learned in countries where the HIV epidemic began much earlier and will institute HIV prevention programs before the epidemic becomes more widespread.

In Western Europe, where HIV has been a public health problem for nearly as long as in the United States, the picture is quite different. As in the United States, nosocomial transmissions have clearly leveled off, and homosexual males and intravenous drug users account for the vast majority of cumulative AIDS cases. The relative importance of these routes varies by country. Homosexual and bisexual transmission are responsible for at least 70% of reported AIDS cases in Denmark, Germany, the Netherlands, Norway, Sweden, and the United Kingdom, whereas IVDU transmission assumes greater importance in Italy (66%) and Spain (63%).

The AIDS cases appearing today, however, represent infections that may have been transmitted 10 or more years ago. WHO projections for the 1990s suggest that the fastest growing HIV transmission category in Europe at present is neither homosexual nor IVDU, but rather the heterosexual partners of persons in those risk groups and their sex partners. Finnish investigators Sirkka-Liisa Valle and Seppo Sarna noted that of 300 cases of HIV infection diagnosed in Finland by mid-May 1990, only 14 were attributed to IVDU, whereas 79 had been acquired through heterosexual contact with an infected partner.

Anneke van den Hoek and colleagues, who studied the sexual behavior of 243 Dutch intravenous drug users, found that whereas HIV and other STDs were common in this population, condom use was not. Among drug-using prostitutes, those who consistently used condoms with their commercial partners were less inclined to do so with private partners, although condom use increased with knowledge of positive serostatus. The researchers concluded that IVDUs are likely to constitute an important source of heterosexual transmission of HIV.

Reports from Belgium, where the incidence of heterosexually transmitted HIV is perhaps the highest in Europe, suggest that encounters with HIV-positive persons from pattern II countries represent another important source of transmission.

Asia. Although HIV was introduced on that continent only recently, the virus is spreading with frightening speed among a number of IVDU and prostitute groups. The most vivid example is in Thailand, where HIV first appeared in the homosexual community in the mid-1980s. Around 1986, it spread to intravenous drug users and was so rapidly disseminated that, by early 1988, the seroprevalence rate among IVDUs in Bangkok had risen to 16%. Today it approaches 50%. The third wave of the epidemic began among prostitutes and their heterosexual partners in the late 1980s. Again, HIV spread very rapidly, with seroprevalence rates rising from under 1% to as high as 40% in some areas over a period of less than two years.

Similar explosive spread of HIV is taking place in India (with nearly 20% of the world's population), where rates of infection in certain prostitute populations have rapidly climbed to 30% or more. Although a survey in southeastern India as early as February 1986 showed that 10% of urban prostitutes were infected, serious national efforts to deal with the epidemic are only now beginning. Poverty, prostitution, widespread STDs, and absence of circumcision in the Hindu population could portend a major HIV epidemic in India during the coming decade. A second focus of HIV spread in India has been found in IVDUs in Manipur in the northeastern part of the country bordering the heroin-producing "Golden Triangle" of Asia. The epidemic of HIV among IVDUs has fanned out from Manipur to Myanmar, northern Thailand, and China.

No cases of AIDS had been reported in China, home of another 20% of the world's population, until 1988, when an IVDU-related outbreak was detected among minority tribesmen in Yunnan Province on the western border of the country, near the Golden Triangle. Sexual transmission of HIV is not expected to pose a major problem in China—although the number of STD cases reported there has been doubling annually since the late 1970s, following the opening of China's borders and increases in internal migration of male workers during the 1970s and 1980s, along with a resurgence of prostitution.

In the Philippines, Indonesia, Malasia, Sri Lanka, Taiwan, Korea, and Singapore, the prevalence of HIV infection among prostitutes has remained surprisingly low, although the potential for a heterosexual HIV epidemic is considered high where extensive commercial sex industries exist. Among the industrialized countries, Japan has been spared to a great extent. So far, the largest proportion of AIDS patients there received blood products before 1986.

In summary, a very conservative WHO estimate is that about half a million cases of HIV infection have occurred in Asia, but some experts believe the number could easily be two or three times greater. Nearly all of these cases have been in India and Thailand. With more than twice the population of sub-Saharan Africa, and a rate of spread comparable to that in Africa in the 1980s, southern Asia could well experience a pandemic during the 1990s bigger than the African pandemic.

Africa. The current situation in sub-Saharan Africa is puzzling in that HIV rates appear to have stabilized in some countries but not others. In Zaire, for example, the infection seems to be leveling off at prevalence rates of around 6% to 7% in the capital, Kinshasa, and at even lower rates in rural areas. In nearby Rwanda, however, HIV rates have continued to climb, and in urban areas of Uganda and Zambia, rates as high as 40% are being reported. Whether these variations reflect regional differences in patterns of sexual activity and sexual networking, prevalence of genital ulcer disease and other STDs, circumcision rates, or some other, unknown factor, has not been established. In light of the considerable correlation between absence of circumcision in some African ethnic groups and high rates of HIV infection and other STDs, interest has been growing in prospective studies of circumcision and acquisition of HIV in high-risk areas.

Although condom promotion and distribution programs have been shown to be helpful in reducing HIV transmission, they have not been implemented in all nations with high HIV prevalence. For example, Uganda, with one of the highest rates of HIV infection in the world—10% of the overall population and much higher in the urban capital, Kampala—has no real condom promotion policy. Where such programs have been implemented, as in Kenya, they have often run up against strong cultural opposition. Men resist efforts of women, including prostitutes, to promote use of condoms for STD prevention. Efforts by female prostitutes to induce barrier protection often tend to be futile. Family planning programs that emphasize other, more effective, contraceptive methods are often reluctant to see condoms promoted for contraception as well as disease prophylaxis. And those programs that do promote condoms for contraception have been nervous about "confusing" the public with dual messages about using condoms for both purposes.

In a study of the factors associated with heterosexual spread of HIV in a large population of office workers in Kinshasa, Robert W. Ryder and co-workers found that married men engaged in a high rate of unprotected extramarital sex with younger, unmarried women and prostitutes. Typically, those who acquired HIV or another STD continued to have unprotected sex with their wives—thereby placing both the wives and any children they might bear at risk of infection. Only 10% of couples used condoms or another form of birth control, and even in this group use was sporadic.

Men who had numerous sex partners and those with histories of both genital ulcer disease and prostitute contact were at significantly higher risk of acquiring HIV. For the workers' wives, an HIV-positive spouse, receipt of a blood transfusion, or history of genital ulcer disease was independently associated with HIV risk. This study underscores the need to coordinate AIDS education in developing countries with aggressive policies promoting condom use and prevention and control of genital ulcer disease and other STDs.

Caribbean and Latin America. As of early 1991, the cumulative total number of cases of HIV infection estimated to have occurred in this region was 1 million, with just over 100,000 cases of AIDS. An estimated 10,000 children have been born with HIV infection.

The countries of the Caribbean subregion have been hard hit by HIV. Nearly everywhere in the region, heterosexual transmission predominates (Figure 2), many women are infected, and pediatric AIDS is having a powerful impact on child mortality. Reported incidence is highest in the Bahamas (38 cases per 100,000 population); however, HIV seroprevalence is believed to be even higher in Haiti and its neighbor, the Dominican Republic.

Haiti shares many of the societal problems that have facilitated transmission of the virus in Africa: grinding poverty, political unrest, lack of educational and employment opportunity, and high rates of prostitution and STDs in general.

Worker migration from one nation to another has promoted spread of the epidemic. For example, movement of farm workers between the

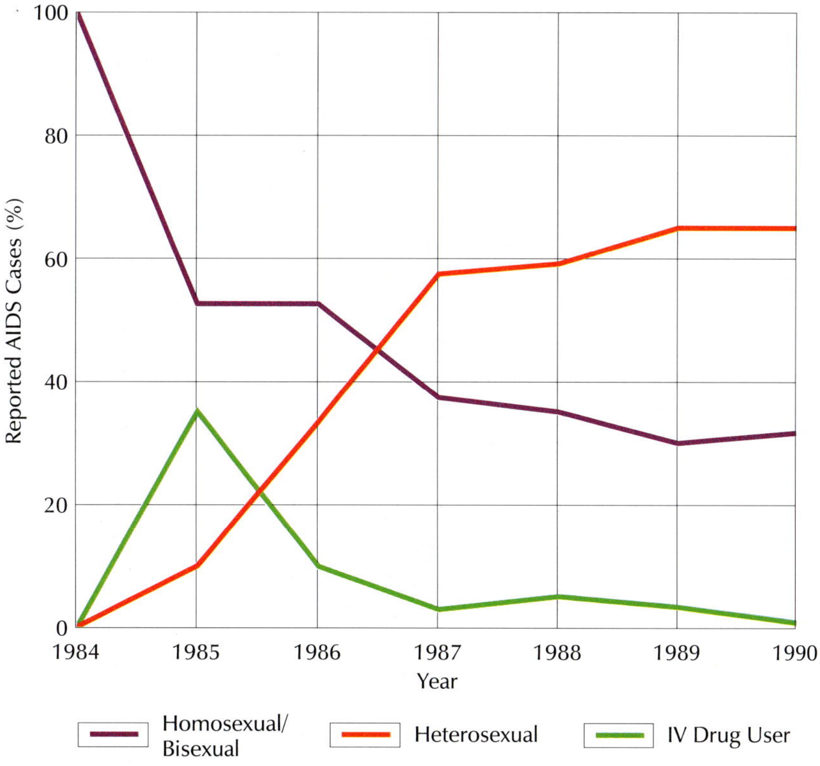

Figure 2 From 1984 to 1990, reported AIDS cases in Caribbean countries underwent a profound shift in distribution according to risk category. Cases identified with homosexual or bisexual contact declined from 100% to 32%, and those involving heterosexual contact rose from 0% to 65%. Except for 1985, intravenous drug users have not been major factors in the disease's spread in the region.

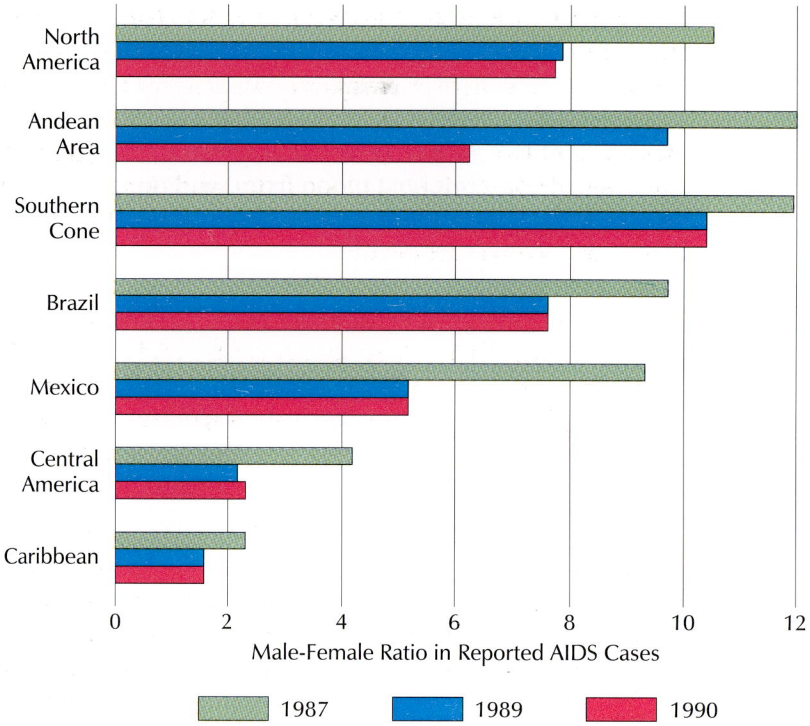

Figure 3 As in North America, AIDS cases reported in most of Latin America and the Caribbean have predominantly involved males and homosexual transmission. But the trend in recent years has been toward a narrowing of male-female ratios, reflecting increases in heterosexual transmission. The changes have ranged from dramatic (e.g., in Andean countries) to gradual (e.g., in Caribbean countries).

Caribbean and southern Florida has encouraged the spread of HIV in both areas. The predominantly male composition of migrant communities, their economic marginality, and their separation from families and isolation from the social mainstream tend to foster contact with prostitutes and transmission of STDs.

In Mexico and most of Central and South America, homosexual activity remains the prevailing mode of HIV transmission—although cases involving heterosexual exposures are increasing at a rapid rate, especially in large urban centers and along the Caribbean coast (Figure 3). A notable feature of the epidemic in this region has been the central role played by bisexual men, who tend to marry and have children while at the same time pursuing an active homosexual life-style. As with IVDUs in Europe, bisexual men form an essential link in the chain of transmission that allows the virus to gain entry into the larger heterosexual population.

In those areas of Western Europe where many IVDUs are infected with HIV, the rate of spread to heterosexual partners has probably been slowed by effective STD control programs and widespread availability of family planning and preventive health services. No such barriers exist in the sprawling slums of Rio de Janeiro, São Paolo, or Mexico City, where the epidemic is fueled by sexually transmitted disease and economic desperation. Prostitutes, including several million homeless children who survive by selling or exchanging sex for food, represent a growing reservoir of HIV. Although rapid progress is being made in blood banking, sale of contaminated blood from paid donors to unlicensed blood banks and inadequate sterilization of blood collection equipment have continued to pose problems.

Relatively fewer AIDS cases have been reported from the Andean region of South America and the countries that make up the continent's southern cone: Chile, Uruguay, Argentina, and Paraguay. Yet the percentage of heterosexual transmissions is increasing there as well. In Chile, for example, 15% of AIDS cases are attributable to heterosexual exposures—roughly two to three times the current U.S. rate.

United States and Canada. By May 1991, 179,694 cases of AIDS had been reported in the United States and more than 4,000 in Canada. The demographics of the epidemic were similar in both countries, with homosexual and bisexual men making up the majority (now roughly 60%) of adult AIDS cases, IVDUs accounting for a sizable minority (now 22% in the United States), and heterosexual contact cases not associated with drug use accounting for approximately 6%. Receipt of contaminated blood or clotting factors accounted for only 2% of AIDS cases in this region in 1990, and fewer than 2% of cases occurred among children under 13. (The CDC estimates that 85% of U.S. AIDS cases are reported, although at least one survey has suggested that reporting in some states may be as low as 60%. In addition, certain population groups—blacks, IVDUs, persons with no known risk factors—tend to be chronically underrepresented in AIDS case estimates.)

Obviously, reported AIDS cases represent only a small percentage of the total number of persons infected with HIV. To determine the actual dimensions of the U.S. epidemic and predict growth patterns, the CDC relies on 1) back-calculation of the number of HIV infections necessary to account for the AIDS cases that have already been reported, and 2) extrapolation from HIV seroprevalence data derived from specific groups, such as Red Cross blood donors, active-duty military personnel, and homosexual men in observed cohorts. On the basis of these analyses, the CDC estimates that 1 million U.S. citizens are currently infected with HIV and that at least 40,000 new HIV infections occur each year among adults and adolescents. Serosurveys of blood specimens from newborns further suggest that 0.05% of all infants born each year in the United States (between 1,500 and 2,000) are infected with the virus.

In the United States, the volume of AIDS cases is disproportionately high among blacks and Hispanics. Blacks make up approximately 12% of the U.S. population but 27% to 30% of diagnosed AIDS cases; Hispanics, who make up 8% of the population, represent 16% to 17% of AIDS cases. The disparity is greatest among women and children: 57% of

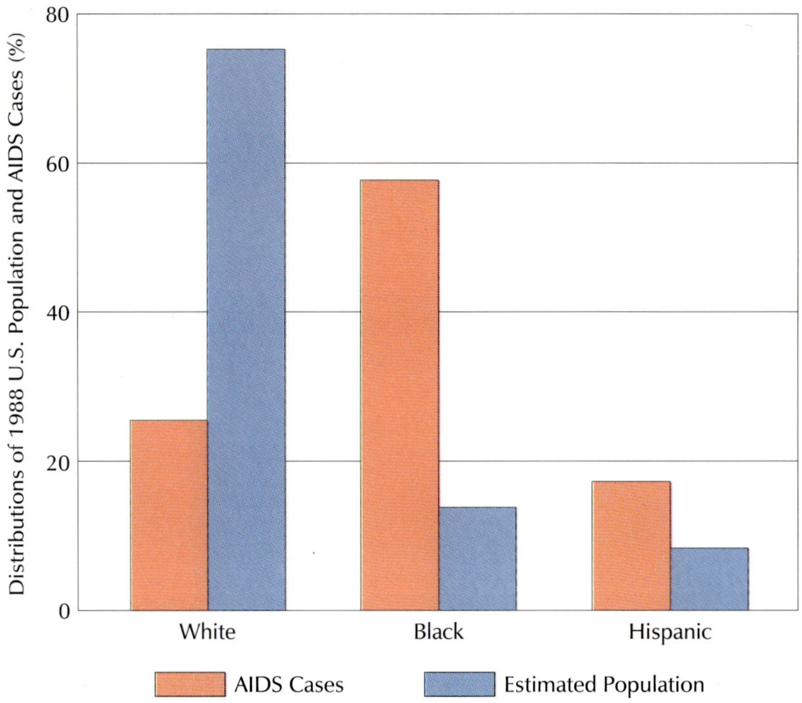

Figure 4 In the United States, AIDS disproportionately affects blacks and Hispanics—especially women and children. Thus, 1988 data show that, whereas whites (75% of the female population) accounted for about 25% of AIDS cases in women, blacks accounted for almost 60% and Hispanics for about 17%. A similar pattern was evident in children (not shown).

women and 54% of children with AIDS are black; 17% of AIDS-affected women and 21% of AIDS-affected children are Hispanic (Figure 4).

With the exception of transfusion recipients and persons with hemophilia, the number of new AIDS cases diagnosed per year in the United States is expected to continue to rise over the next several years in each of the principal transmission groups: homosexual and bisexual men, IVDUs, persons infected heterosexually, and children infected perinatally. However, as shown in Table 3, the relative contribution of each of these groups to the total number of AIDS cases is clearly changing in response to shifts in transmission dynamics.

One major trend that has already become apparent is the leveling off of AIDS diagnoses among homosexual and bisexual men, especially in large cities such as New York, San Francisco, and Los Angeles. Whereas AIDS diagnoses rose sharply in the years between 1981 and 1987 for all groups of homosexual and bisexual men, the curve subsequently began to flatten for white homosexual and bisexual men who did not use intravenous drugs. Not affected by the shift were homosexual men who were black or Hispanic, or men who used IV drugs.

A number of explanations for this trend have been offered: First,

Table 3. Projected Numbers of AIDS Cases by Transmission Group,* United States, 1989–1993

Year	*Homosexual and Bisexual Men*		*Heterosexual Male and Female*		
	Not Intravenous Drug Users	*Intravenous Drug Users*	*Intravenous Drug Users*	*Heterosexual Transmission*	*Perinatal Transmission*
1989	26,000–28,000	2,600–2,800	11,000	2,600–2,900	1,000–1,100
1990	29,000–31,000	2,700–3,000	13,000–14,000	3,700–4,000	1,300–1,500
1991	30,000–38,000	2,600–3,400	14,000–18,000	4,800–6,100	1,600–2,200
1992	30,000–44,000	2,500–3,600	16,000–23,000	6,100–8,800	2,100–3,100
1993	30,000–48,000	2,400–3,800	17,000–27,000	7,600–12,200	2,600–4,100
Cumulative total through 1993† 11,000–14,000	219,000–262,000	21,000–25,000	95,000–118,000	29,000–38,000	

* Projections are adjusted for unreported diagnoses of AIDS by adding 18% to projections obtained from reported cases (corresponding to 85% of all diagnosed cases being reported: 1/0.85=1.18) and rounded (to the nearest 1,000 for the first and third groups, and to nearest 100 for the other three groups).

† Rounded to the nearest 1,000. Includes the following numbers of cases estimated to have been diagnosed through 1988: 74,000 among homosexual and bisexual men who are not intravenous drug users (IVDUs); 8,600 among homosexual and bisexual men who are IVDUs; 25,000 among heterosexual male and female IVDUs; 4,200 attributed to heterosexual transmission; and 1,900 attributed to perinatal transmission. (Adapted from MMWR, November 30, 1990)

"safer sex" campaigns have met with notable success among white homosexual and bisexual men but with considerably less success among black and Hispanic homosexual and bisexual men and IVDUs. Second, use of antiviral and other drug treatments is much higher among whites than among minorities because of such issues as treatment cost, access to transportation to acquire treatment, and degree of comfort with the medical system. Third, the minority populations at greatest risk for HIV include a high proportion of persons of low socioeconomic status with multiple risk factors—i.e., homosexual and bisexual men who share intravenous needles, engage in prostitute sex, or have other STDs.

A second major trend has been the steady rise in heterosexually acquired AIDS cases, from fewer than 1% of all cases in 1983 to more than 6% by the beginning of 1990 through June 1991 (Table 4). Most of these cases have resulted from primary contacts with intravenous drug users. However, as the Finnish example demonstrated, more extensive spread to tertiary contacts may simply be a matter of time. Although dwarfed in terms of absolute numbers by homosexual and IVDU transmission, heterosexual contact is now the fastest-growing category of HIV transmission in the United States.

Table 4. Percentage of Heterosexually Acquired AIDS Cases by Quarter of Diagnosis, 1983–1990*

1983	1984	1985	1986	1987	1988	1989	1990
0.88%	1.43%	1.78%	2.11%	2.84%	3.64%	4.64%	5.75%
1.34%	1.13%	2.01%	2.59%	3.30%	4.33%	4.89%	6.24%
1.01%	1.55%	1.91%	2.65%	3.57%	4.36%	5.04%	6.16%
0.79%	1.55%	2.40%	2.62%	3.58%	4.17%	4.95%	6.26%

Like IVDU-related AIDS, heterosexual AIDS is disproportionately a problem of urban minorities. The cumulative incidence per million population is more than 11 times greater for black and Hispanic women than for white women. Among men, the cumulative AIDS incidence is more than 10 times greater for blacks and 4 times greater for Hispanics than for whites. Similarly, the female-male ratio of heterosexually acquired AIDS in the United States is higher for blacks (2.1:1) and Hispanics (4.3:1) than for whites (1.9:1).

The distribution of heterosexual AIDS cases within the U.S. population closely parallels that of other heterosexually transmitted infections. Although the overall incidence of gonorrhea has been declining since the mid-1970s, the incidence in the black population rose sharply between 1984 and 1986. Profiles of patients seen during a penicillin-resistant gonorrhea outbreak that occurred in Seattle in 1986–1987 were remarkably consistent: Most were heterosexual black men and women, and more than 80% had histories of recent prostitution, sex with prostitutes, use of IV drugs or crack cocaine, or sex exchanged for crack cocaine.

The resurgence of infectious syphilis in the minority population has been even more dramatic, especially in major cities, where it has been closely linked to the exchange of sex for crack cocaine. In 1987, incidence rates for early syphilis in the United States were 25 times higher among black men and 12 times higher among Hispanic men than among white men. They were 31 times higher among black women and 8 times higher among Hispanic women than among white women.

Chancroid was rare in the United States between the close of World War II and the mid-1980s. Then it, too, reappeared in minority and migrant-labor populations. In 1984, there were 665 chancroid cases in the United States and in 1989, there were 4,714. Other sexually transmitted infections—including those caused by *C. trachomatis*, herpes simplex virus type 2, human papillomavirus, and hepatitis B virus—have also risen to epidemic levels in the U.S. population. In addition to the independent damage they cause, several of the STDs increase the efficiency of HIV transmission and, reciprocally, their spread is also promoted by HIV.

The association between the resurgence of STDs and the introduction of crack cocaine into the Caribbean and the United States from Latin America in the mid-1980s is inescapable. Data from the National Centers for Drug Abuse show a steady rise in emergency room admissions for crack use from 1985 until mid-1990. Income generated by the drug trade radically altered the social structure of inner-city communities by placing large sums of money in the hands of teenagers and young adults who lacked job skills or professional role models.

Adolescent girls and young women, many of them not previously prostitutes, began to traffic in large numbers of sexual contacts to support their crack habit. Whereas veteran prostitutes in today's climate—particularly those not addicted to drugs—tend to use condoms with their paying contacts (although less frequently with private contacts), crack-addicted prostitutes do not. Lack of barrier protection thus intensified the relationship between STDs, HIV, and crack.

The higher birthrates of U.S. minority populations as compared with that of the white population may be an additional contributing factor in the rapid spread of HIV among minorities. The age pyramid of our urban poor—with its bulge representing children, adolescents, and young adults—is not dissimilar to the age pyramids of pattern II areas in which heterosexual AIDS is already endemic. Not only are young people more sexually active than older adults, they also tend to ignore the consequences of high-risk behavior of any type. Data from the homosexual community suggests that while safer-sex practices have been adopted by the majority of adult men, a significant percentage of gay teenagers are engaging in unprotected sex—and acquiring STDs, including HIV infection.

A Domestic Crisis

Rising rates of HIV and other heterosexually transmitted diseases in our cities have created a massive demand for diagnostic and treatment services. During the past 15 years, federal, state, and municipal spending for public health services have not kept up with the growing need in many areas. One result is that STD clinics that formerly accepted patients until late in the afternoon often were forced to close their doors early in the morning. Although patients who cannot be seen are routinely invited to come back the following day, many become discouraged or irritated by the wait and fail to return. At a time when a growing proportion of those who acquire and spread STDs are becoming harder and harder to reach through partner notification, it is ironic that we are turning such patients away when they do show up for care.

A principal barrier to serving persons needing diagnosis and treatment has been failure to provide sufficient numbers of clinicians to see patients in public STD clinics. The facilities have also been allowed to deteriorate throughout the country. Federal funding for STD control so far is not allowed to be used for clinical care, and local support has not been forthcoming. Denial of appropriations for STD diagnosis and treatment has been explained away on the basis that management of existing cases is of less long-term importance than primary prevention. Although this may be true in other contexts, it is extremely shortsighted when dealing with communicable diseases. When such a disease is curable, primary care *is* a form of primary prevention, because it removes the pathogen from circulation.

In a survey conducted in 1989, 19 out of 23 public STD clinics in the United States reported one or more features of the pattern of delayed care just described. The situation appears even more shameful in light of the effectiveness of STD control programs undertaken by Canada, as well as by Japan, Australia, New Zealand, and virtually all of the countries of Western Europe. In none of those countries (with isolated exceptions) has gonorrhea, syphilis, or chancroid resurfaced, as they have in the United States.

Obviously, culturally sensitive health education programs on avoidance of illicit drugs and promiscuity are essential. The success of safer-sex campaigns in reducing the spread of HIV among white homosexual men is evidence that public health education can work. Its failure among blacks and Hispanics and IVDUs and their heterosexual partners may reflect the fact that health education programs have gotten under way more slowly in these groups or that different educational tools are required for different populations.

More federal and state spending on primary care for the sexually transmitted diseases that fuel the HIV epidemic is another absolute requirement. *C. trachomatis* infection is an example: Studies have shown that chlamydial infection is a major cause of infertility in women, that it may cause premature births, and that perinatal transfer can result in infant pneumonia. It has also been associated with increased transmission efficiency of HIV infection, as discussed earlier.

The direct and indirect medical costs of dealing with *C. trachomatis* infection were estimated at $1.5 billion a year in the mid-1980s and are probably considerably higher today. Yet, although comprehensive programs to control chlamydial infection have been formulated by health care policymakers, only in rare cases have they been implemented by local health departments or practicing physicians.

Patients with AIDS are living longer today than in the early years of the epidemic, and they require skilled care by local physicians and community clinic staff. The impression that most persons with HIV infection can be cared for only by specialists in a hospital setting is seriously misguided. In addition, as these patients remain active longer, their potential for spreading the virus could increase, intensifying the need for counseling regarding safer sex and avoidance of illicit IV drugs.

Of course, the real solution to the evolving health crisis in cities lies in societal change to reduce the glaring inequities that lie at its root. Poverty, social dislocation, and lack of educational and professional opportunity leave vulnerable young people prey to drugs, prostitution, and HIV. Treat the causes of these inequities, and you treat the disease.

SELECTED READING

Aral SO, Holmes KK: Sexually transmitted diseases in the AIDS era. Sci Am 264(2):62, 1991

Chin J: Current and future dimensions of the HIV/AIDS pandemic in women and children. Lancet 336:221, 1990

Hartgers C et al: The impact of the needle and syringe-exchange programme in Amsterdam on injecting risk behaviour. AIDS 3:571, 1989

Holmes KK et al: The increasing frequency of heterosexually acquired AIDS in the United States, 1983–88. Am J Public Health 80:858, 1990

May RM, Anderson RM: Transmission dynamics of HIV infection. Nature 326:137, 1987

Quinn TC, Narain JP, Zacarias FRK: AIDS in the Americas: A public health priority for the region. AIDS 4:709, 1990

Ryder RW et al: Heterosexual transmission of HIV-1 among employees and their spouses at two large businesses in Zaire. AIDS 4:725, 1990

Stoneburner RL et al: The epidemic of AIDS and HIV-1 infection among heterosexuals in New York City. AIDS 4:99, 1990

van den Hoek JAR, van Haastrecht HJA, Coutinho RA: Heterosexual behavior of intravenous drug users in Amsterdam: Implications for the AIDS epidemic. AIDS 4:449, 1990

4 Current Status of HIV Therapy: I. Antiretroviral Agents

DANIEL F. HOTH, JR., MAUREEN W. MYERS, *and*
DANIEL S. STEIN
National Institute of Allergy and Infectious Diseases

After less than a decade, the face of human immunodeficiency virus infection in the United States has changed. In the early 1980s, most patients presented with advanced HIV infection complicated by opportunistic infections or malignancies. Today, more patients are being diagnosed at the stage of early, asymptomatic HIV infection. With this change, management of HIV-infected patients has evolved two strategies: one directed against the virus itself to delay or prevent progression of disease and one to prevent or treat opportunistic infections and malignancies. The first strategy is the subject of this discussion. The second strategy will be addressed in part II of the discussion on opportunistic infection therapy.

Although opportunistic diseases loom larger in the day-to-day management of advanced HIV infection, the basic strategy against HIV disease must, of course, focus on the virus itself. A major international effort has been mobilized to develop new agents for treating HIV infection, and that effort is beginning to produce results. Many new antiretroviral compounds are in various stages of preclinical or clinical evaluation. In the United States, much of the clinical work is being carried out by the AIDS Clinical Trials Group (ACTG), which comprises investigators from 52 medical centers and operates under the auspices of the Division of AIDS of the National Institute of Allergy and Infectious Diseases (NIAID). There is also a substantial commitment of resources by the pharmaceutical industry to discovery, development, and clinical testing.

Antiretroviral agents can target any of several steps in the viral life cycle. Potential points of attack include the attachment of virions to the host cell membrane, reverse transcription of RNA to DNA, transcription of viral cDNA integrated into host-cell DNA, translation, and assembly of viral genomic RNA and proteins into virions (Figure 1).

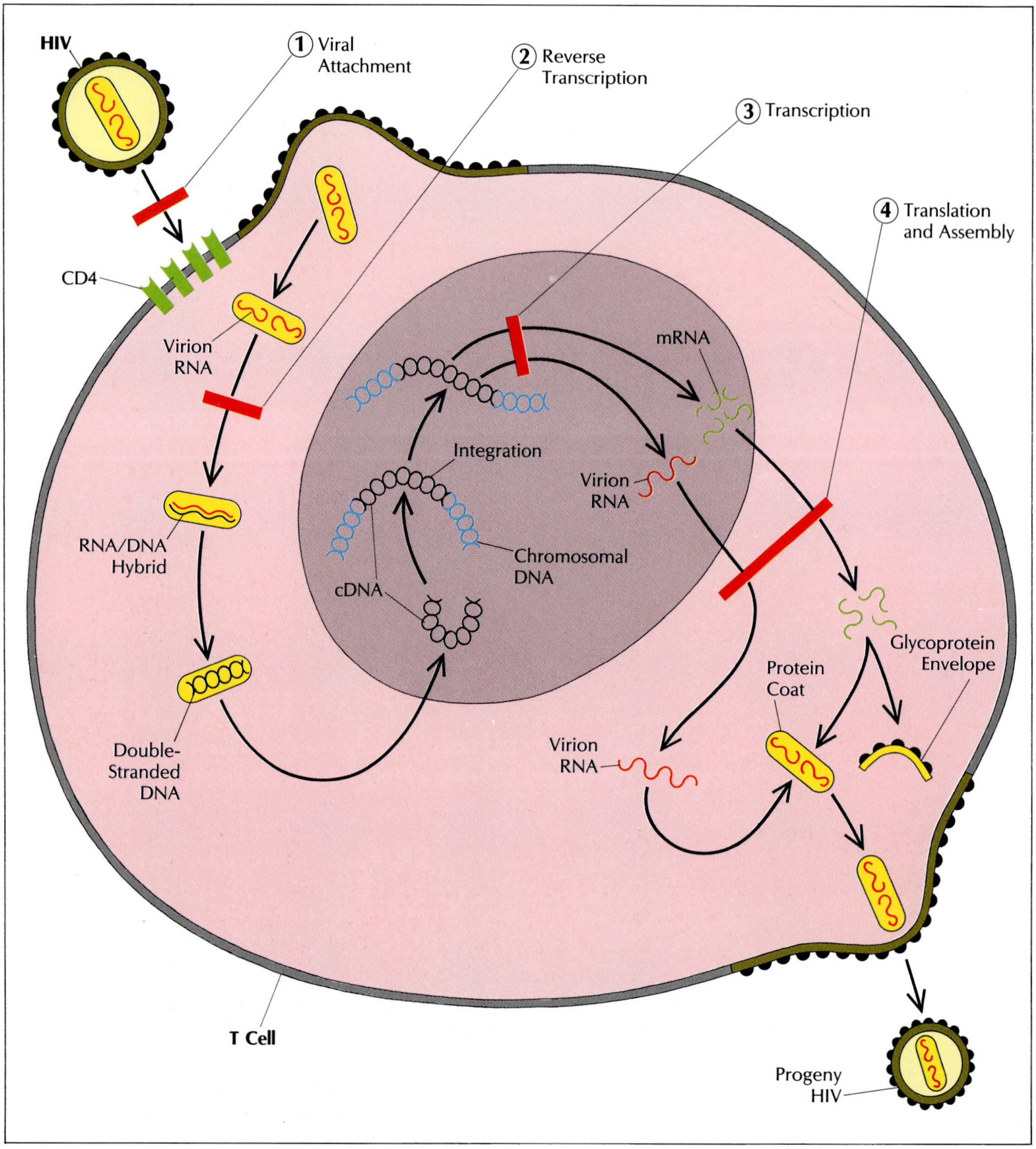

Figure 1 Antiretroviral agents may inhibit any of several steps in the HIV life cycle: 1) attachment to host cell membrane, 2) reverse transcription of viral RNA to DNA, 3) transcription of viral cDNA integrated into host cell DNA, or 4) translation and assembly of viral RNA and proteins. Notably, reverse transcription is inhibited by zidovudine.

Zidovudine

Zidovudine (3'-azido-3'-deoxythymidine)—formerly AZT—was the first antiretroviral drug approved by the Food and Drug Administration. A thymidine analogue that replaces the 3' hydroxyl group with an azido moiety, zidovudine is phosphorylated by cellular enzymes to a 5'-triphosphate form that competes with natural thymidine triphosphate for binding to HIV reverse transcriptase, thereby inhibiting the rate of viral DNA synthesis. The 5'-triphosphate form can also act as an alternate substrate for reverse transcriptase and be incorporated into the growing DNA chain. Since it has no 3' hydroxyl group for attachment of the next nucleotide, chain elongation stops, and production of a DNA copy of viral RNA—necessary for integration into host cell DNA—is inhibited.

Zidovudine is not a cure for HIV infection, but it delays progression of immunodeficiency and onset of symptoms in early disease. In later disease, it decreases the frequency and severity of opportunistic infections, partially ameliorates the neuropsychiatric dysfunction often seen in AIDS patients, and prolongs survival. Early use of zidovudine and PCP prophylaxis has slowed the increase in the number of AIDS cases to below that originally projected several years ago. In addition, recent epidemiologic evidence supports prolongation of survival by this approach.

Zidovudine produces improvement in immunologic status as measured by increases in CD4+ T-lymphocyte counts and skin-test reactivity, response to vaccination, and interferon production. Antiviral activity in patients is indicated by a decrease in quantitative measures of both plasma- and cell-associated virus and serum levels of HIV p24 core antigen. Because of the unusual urgency for development of new antiretroviral agents, CD4 and p24 levels are often used as surrogates for clinical efficacy. It has not yet been conclusively demonstrated, however, that surrogate markers can replace clinical end points. Diminishing CD4 levels have been definitively associated with disease progression and decreased survival, but treatment-induced changes in CD4 levels have not yet been correlated with improved disease outcome.

On the other hand, current data suggest that p24 antigen may in fact not be useful as a surrogate for drug-related clinical benefit. Levels of circulating p24 antigen are considered a measure of the intensity of viral replication, and in general, p24 levels tend to increase as infection progresses and to drop in response to effective therapy. Those changes are neither dramatic nor completely consistent, however. Many patients—especially those with early HIV disease, but some late-stage patients as well—do not show p24 antigen, and many study subjects who have shown clinical improvement have had no change or have had increases in p24 levels. By definition, a marker that does not consistently parallel the progression of disease cannot be consistently useful as a surrogate for response to treatment.

Research interest is currently focusing on the reproducible quantitation of whole-virus levels in serum and cells as a direct measure of antiretroviral drug effect. Because of the technical demands of the procedure and unresolved questions about specimen processing, measurement of both plasma- and cell-associated viremia has no clinical utility at present. Such assays have, however, been used in phase I studies to measure antiviral activity of agents under study. If the assays do eventually enter clinical use, logical applications would be for monitoring antiretroviral drug activity and deciding when to change or start therapy. Measurement of all of the immunologic and virologic markers that we have discussed depends on a stringent quality-control program to reduce variability, both within and between laboratories, for optimal utility.

Clinical benefits from zidovudine may be apparent as early as six weeks after initiation of therapy. In 1986, Margaret A. Fischl and colleagues enrolled 281 subjects with AIDS or AIDS-related complex in a placebo-controlled study of zidovudine. An interim analysis at six months revealed that the zidovudine group had not only fewer opportunistic infections but also a significant survival advantage.

Because all placebo subjects were then offered zidovudine, long-term direct comparison between treated and placebo groups is not available. At follow-up, however, analysis of 229 of the subjects showed that patients with AIDS who had initially been randomized to zidovudine lived longer than those who were originally randomized to placebo and then switched to zidovudine (Figure 2). Mortality did increase over time in zidovudine recipients, and it was particularly evident after the first year of therapy. Other studies have indicated similar findings.

Toxicity from zidovudine was common in the study subjects. Adverse reactions tended to occur early in the course of therapy—the major one being bone marrow suppression, as indicated by granulocytopenia and anemia. The first episode of granulocytopenia typically occurred within the first four months of therapy and responded to lowering of the dose or temporary interruption of the drug regimen. Serious anemia was most common during the first two months of therapy and typically could be managed the same way, although approximately half of affected subjects required red blood cell transfusion.

The study also showed that a possible late-developing adverse reaction to zidovudine is myopathy. Its incidence and severity are unknown, but severe myopathy appears to be related to duration of zidovudine therapy and its effect on muscle mitochondria. Similarly, late hepatotoxicity may occur, but it is rare.

The next step was to evaluate a lower dose. The ACTG (protocol 002) compared two zidovudine dosage regimens in 524 AIDS patients after a first episode of *Pneumocystis carinii* pneumonia: the then-standard daily dose of 1,500 mg, and a daily dose of 1,200 mg for four weeks followed by 600 mg. The lower dose proved equally effective in terms of survival as well as frequency and severity of opportunistic infections, particularly PCP. Not surprisingly, it also proved less toxic. Serious anemia and

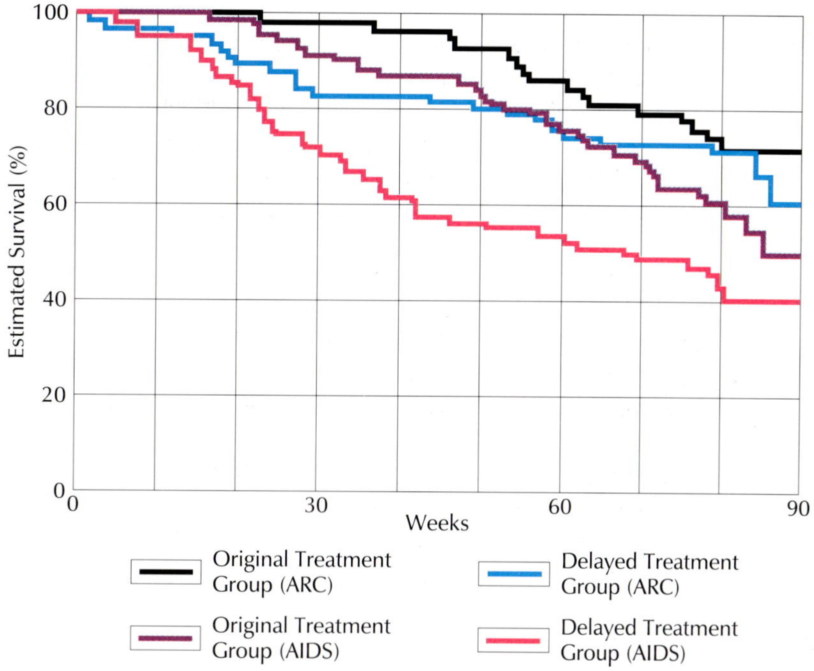

Figure 2 After six months of a placebo-controlled trial of zidovudine therapy in 281 patients with AIDS or AIDS-related complex, a survival advantage with zidovudine was apparent, and all placebo subjects were then offered the drug. Subsequent analysis revealed an advantage with early treatment. Estimated survival was greater in AIDS patients originally randomized to zidovudine, compared with that in AIDS patients whose treatment was delayed. The negative effect of delaying treatment was less prominent among patients with ARC.

neutropenia developed less often and later in the low-dose group: 29% had a hemoglobin concentration of less than 8 gm/dl, compared with 39% in the standard treatment group; 37% had neutrophil counts below 750, compared with 51% in the standard treatment group.

Other studies supported the use of zidovudine earlier in HIV infection. In a double-blind placebo-controlled trial of zidovudine in less immunosuppressed (CD4 counts of 200 to 800) but mildly symptomatic patients (protocol 016), the ACTG found that the drug delayed progression of disease in subjects with CD4 counts of less than 500 (Figure 3). The progression rate was low for those with CD4 counts of 500 or more, but there were too few subjects in that group to provide definitive evidence of benefit from zidovudine. A daily dose of 1,200 mg was used in the trial.

In theory, the earlier zidovudine is started in HIV infection, the better tolerated and more effective it should be, because the patient is less seriously ill and has a more intact immune system and a smaller viral load. In fact, among mildly symptomatic subjects receiving zidovudine in protocol 016, the rate of significant neutropenia was only 4% and that of anemia only 5%.

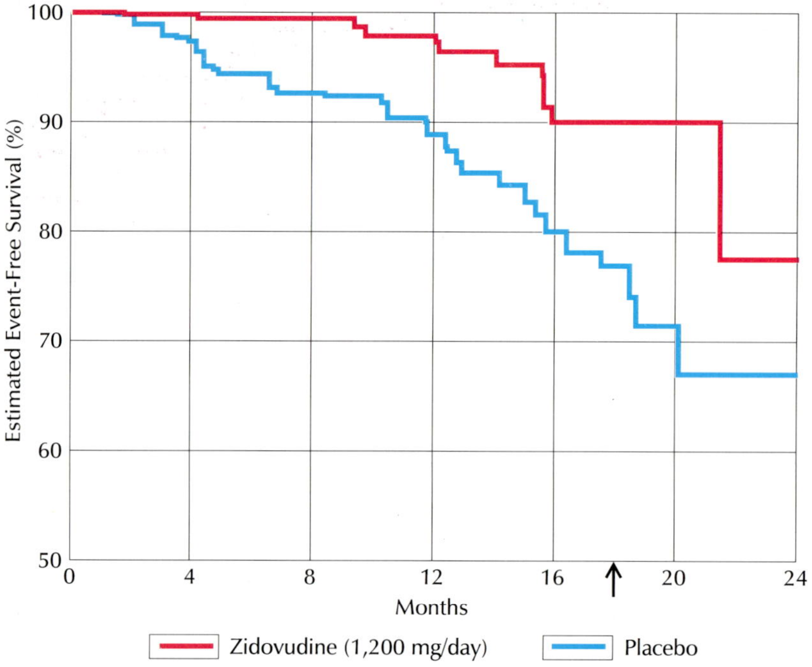

Figure 3 In patients with mildly symptomatic HIV infection and CD4 counts of less than 500, treatment with zidovudine delayed progression of disease. At 18 months (arrow), estimated event-free survival in patients randomized to the drug was 90%, compared with 76% in those randomized to a placebo.

The logical culmination was the performance of studies in asymptomatic patients. An ACTG study (protocol 019) reported by Paul A. Volberding and colleagues demonstrated benefits from zidovudine in asymptomatic subjects, and at a markedly lower dose. In subjects with CD4 counts below 500, a three-arm comparison of placebo and zidovudine in daily doses of 500 and 1,500 mg showed that both doses equally delayed disease progression (Figure 4). Severe side effects were less frequent than in other studies involving subjects with AIDS or symptomatic HIV infection. As one would expect, however, hematologic toxicity was more frequent in the 1,500-mg zidovudine group than in the others. The incidence of severe anemia (hemoglobin < 8 gm/dl), for example, was 6.3%, compared with 1.1% in the 500-mg group; no patient given the lower dose required transfusion for anemia. In the 500-mg group, nausea was the only toxic effect seen more frequently than in patients given the placebo.

When the study revealed a significant early benefit, a Data and Safety Monitoring Board recommended that all placebo patients be offered zidovudine—this only two years after the study had started and with a median follow-up of about one year. The researchers cautioned that their study provided no information about the possible long-term benefit or safety of zidovudine. The study stratum of subjects with a CD4 count of less than 500 closed October 31, 1991, and it is currently undergoing

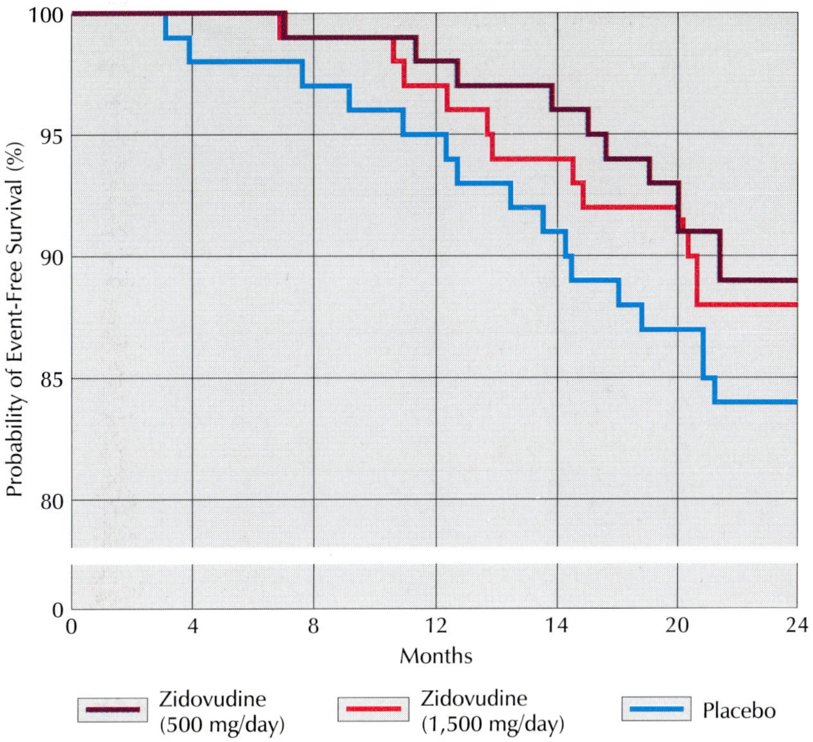

Figure 4 In a placebo-controlled trial of 500 or 1,500 mg/day of zidovudine, 1,338 patients with asymptomatic HIV infection and CD4 counts of less than 500 were followed for up to two years. As judged by the frequency with which AIDS or AIDS-related complex was diagnosed, both low-dose and high-dose zidovudine delayed events in the progression of disease.

analysis. This should yield useful information about long-term therapy and the differential effects of early, compared with later, initiation of therapy. The patients with CD4 counts greater than 500 continue in the double-blind study. It is hoped that this group will help answer the all-important question of whether very early treatment is beneficial.

On the basis of those two trials, in March 1990 the FDA expanded the indications for zidovudine to include asymptomatic and mildly symptomatic HIV infection in patients with CD4 counts below 500. In addition, the FDA lowered the approved dose to 500 mg daily for such asymptomatic patients.

In a recent study, the VA Cooperative Studies Group called into question whether the initiation of antiretroviral therapy in symptomatic patients with CD4 counts of less than 500 affected survival. The study showed a significant slowing in progression to AIDS of the zidovudine group (1,500 mg per day) over the placebo group, consonant with earlier studies, but with no difference in survival. However, a number of subsequent epidemiologic and clinical trials have shown evidence of a survival advantage with the use of antiretroviral therapy and PCP prophylaxis. The ongoing analyses of the long-term follow-up of ACTG 016 and 019 should yield important additional information about the benefits and toxicities of early zidovudine therapy.

The European CONCORDE trial, which is similar in design to ACTG 019 but with survival as the end point, is under way and may eventually be the definitive study in settling the issue of survival advantage with early antiretroviral therapy. Two recent investigations have demonstrated the benefit of antiretroviral therapy in minorities and women to be similar to those observed previously in other studies that mostly involved white men.

The minimum daily dose of zidovudine has not yet been defined, but two intriguing, although not definitive, studies have been published. ACTG protocol 010, which was intended to evaluate whether zidovudine and acyclovir have a synergistic effect against HIV in vivo, compared 300-mg, 600-mg, and 1,500-mg daily doses of zidovudine with and without 4.8 gm of acyclovir. The researchers found no evidence of synergism between the two drugs, but they did find evidence of an antiviral effect from the lowest dose of zidovudine. The significance of the finding is much less secure than those of other zidovudine studies, however, because the number of subjects involved was small: 67 overall, with 28 in the low-dose group.

The Nordic Medical Research Council recently completed a double-blind comparative study of 400 mg (N=160), 800 mg (N=158), and 1,200 mg (N=156) of zidovudine administered in divided doses four times daily. There were no differences in mortality, new AIDS-defining events (though there was a trend toward such events in the 800- and 1,200-mg groups), quality of life scores, or CD4 count changes. The withdrawal of zidovudine for moderate or severe adverse reactions increased with dose: 58%, 63%, and 71% for the 400-, 800-, and 1,200-mg groups, respectively ($p = .01$). Because 500 mg per day is well tolerated, and there is a substantial data base supporting its use, that dose should remain the standard of practice. Nevertheless, further studies of very low daily doses are warranted.

Therapeutic Guidelines

The availability of effective early antiretroviral treatment heightens the importance of early diagnosis of HIV infection, before the onset of symptoms. Since immune status is the primary determinant for starting zidovudine therapy, and the CD4 count is the primary marker of this parameter in HIV infection, a consensus panel convened by the NIAID recommended that a baseline CD4 count be obtained at the time of diagnosis (Figure 5). Patients with CD4 counts over 600 should be monitored every six months. The counts should be repeated every three to four months for patients with CD4 counts of 500 to 600, or with onset of symptoms of HIV infection or other significant clinical deterioration (e.g., thrush, hairy leukoplakia, unintended weight loss, persistent diarrhea, fever, and sweating).

Figure 5. Management Guidelines for HIV-Infected Patients

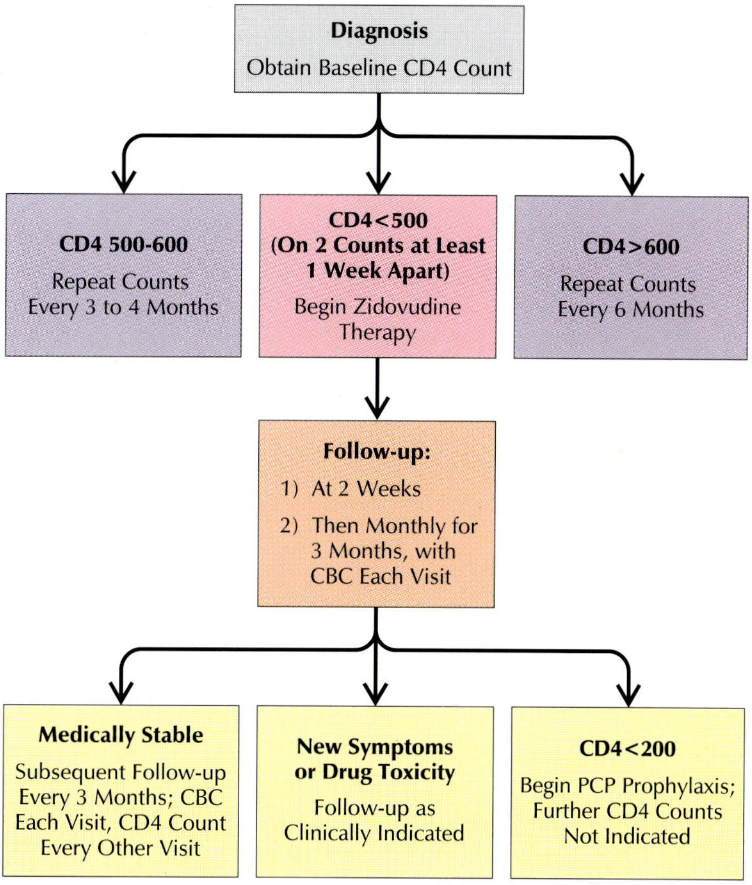

Therapy with zidovudine, 500 mg daily, is recommended for both symptomatic and asymptomatic patients with CD4 counts below 500. For patients with initial values close to 500 (plus or minus 100), the count should be repeated before starting zidovudine. CD4 counts can be transiently altered by many conditions, such as acute viral infections, and variations of as much as 20% are common. Optimally, two consecutive CD4 counts below 500 should be obtained, at least one week apart, before initiation of therapy.

A follow-up visit should be scheduled two weeks after institution of therapy to identify possible side effects from zidovudine and afford the patient an opportunity to express concerns and review information previously discussed. Patients whose condition is clinically stable may be scheduled for subsequent follow-up visits at three-month intervals. More frequent visits are indicated for patients who experience significant adverse events or symptoms that suggest clinical deterioration.

At initiation of zidovudine therapy, a baseline blood cell count with differential and blood chemistry values should be obtained. Abnormal laboratory results should be followed closely. Complete blood counts may be done monthly for the first three months of treatment and every three months thereafter. More frequent monitoring is recommended for patients with abnormal baseline study results or clinical deterioration. Hemoglobin levels less than 8 gm/dl or granulocyte counts of less than 750 indicate serious hematologic toxicity. In that event, zidovudine should be stopped and reinstituted at a lower dose once the abnormalities resolve.

Some clinicians continue treatment at a lower dose (300 mg) in the face of transfusion-dependent anemia; they may use a lower neutrophil threshold for dose adjustment. Other options are to use cytokines for bone marrow stimulation or to switch to didanosine (ddI). Because of possible drug interactions, patients taking medications for treatment of opportunistic infections must be monitored more frequently for toxicity and may require temporary withdrawal of zidovudine. It is unclear at present whether or when zidovudine should be discontinued in favor of other treatment if new disease symptoms arise or laboratory markers change.

Limitations of Zidovudine

Toxicity. With the use of zidovudine in lower doses and earlier in HIV infection, severe toxic reactions to the drug have decreased dramatically. Zidovudine intolerance is still a problem in a small minority of patients, however, particularly those with full-blown AIDS. A possible therapeutic intervention for hematologic toxicity from zidovudine is the addition of cytokines, such as erythropoietin, granulocyte colony-stimulating factor (G-CSF), or granulocyte-macrophage colony-stimulating factor (GM-CSF), in order to stimulate the inhibited bone marrow to increase cellular production.

Resistance. A critical but unanswered question is whether six months to a year of zidovudine therapy can result in the selection of HIV strains that are resistant to the drug. In 15 patients with AIDS or symptomatic HIV infection treated for at least six months, Brendan A. Larder and colleagues at Wellcome Research Laboratories in England and Douglas D. Richman of the University of California, San Diego, documented HIV isolates with greatly reduced in vitro sensitivity to zidovudine, as indicated by reduced ability to inhibit syncytial plaque formation. The isolates showed cross-resistance to only one other antiretroviral agent, azidouridine (AZdU) (more about it below). The appearance of resistant isolates did not herald any sudden or rapid clinical deterioration, however.

Subsequent small studies have examined the association of zidovudine susceptibility with CD4 count decline or clinical events. In general, the isolates with decreased susceptibility are found in patients with disease progression. However, common problems in these studies are the use of post hoc analysis and baseline clinical differences between comparison groups, such as viral load, that preclude demonstration of causation. The incidence of in vitro resistance is significantly less likely in asymptomatic patients with high CD4 counts than in patients with AIDS and low CD4 counts. This suggests that zidovudine treatment of early HIV infection is less likely to produce in vitro resistance than it is in late disease. Specific mutations in HIV-1 reverse transcriptase are associated with resistance to zidovudine as well as ddI, zalcitabine (ddC), foscarnet, and non-nucleoside analogue reverse transcriptase inhibitors. At present, no clinical decisions should be based solely on considerations of resistance. Prospective blinded studies to evaluate resistance and the interaction with virologic, immunologic, and clinical events are currently under way.

Limited efficacy. The principal limitation of zidovudine is that its palliative effect is not sustained, but the optimal duration of therapy with this drug is not known. Despite these limitations, recent evidence from the United States, Europe, and Australia suggests that treatment is having an impact on the course of the epidemic and that zidovudine is a key factor.

Beyond Zidovudine

Although many questions remain about optimizing use of zidovudine, improving the treatment of HIV infection will certainly require new agents, to be used either in combination with or instead of zidovudine. These agents can be categorized according to the stage of viral replication they affect.

Nucleoside analogues. The largest number of promising agents currently in clinical trials can be found in this class of antiviral agents, which includes zidovudine. Although these agents inhibit HIV replication by slightly different mechanisms, all are nucleoside analogues that lack the 3' hydroxyl group and share a common target, HIV reverse transcriptase. The agents include ddI, ddC, statvudine (D4T), AZdU, and 2'-deoxy-3'-thiacytidine (3TC).

ddI. This purine was the second antiretroviral agent to receive FDA approval with an indication for patients who were failing or unable to tolerate zidovudine. In vitro, ddI is less toxic than zidovudine and has significant antiviral activity. Although the plasma half-life of ddI is short (1.3 hours), the active moiety has a prolonged intracellular half-life, which allows twice-daily dosing.

In early clinical trials (including patients with AIDS or symptomatic HIV infection) Samuel Broder and colleagues at the National Cancer Institute, and subsequently others elsewhere, showed that ddI produced significant decreases in serum p24 levels and increases in CD4 counts, in some cases for as long as 40 weeks. Clinical improvement or weight gain was also observed. The major side effects were painful peripheral neuropathy and pancreatitis, which is more likely to occur at higher doses or with once-a-day administration. Dose-related hematologic toxicity was not seen.

The first reported controlled study of the clinical efficacy of ddI was ACTG 116B/117. Early data from this study showing the drug's effect on CD4 counts and from phase I trials were the basis for FDA approval of ddI. The study comprised patients who had completed at least 16 weeks of zidovudine (the median was 13.9 months) randomized to continue zidovudine (N=304), or switched to ddI at either 500 mg daily (N=298) or 750 mg daily (N=311). At entry, the median CD4 counts were between 84 and 98 for the treatment groups, of which 29% to 33% had counts below 50 and about 40% were p24 antigenemic at baseline.

The principal clinical finding was a significantly lower incidence of new AIDS events or death for the 500-mg ddI arm, compared with the zidovudine arm. There was no significant difference for the 750-mg ddI arm, compared with the zidovudine arm. There were no significant differences in overall survival or clinical events among the subgroups of AIDS patients. Pancreatitis was significantly more likely with 750 mg of ddI (13%), compared with 500 mg of ddI (7%) or zidovudine (3%). In contrast to the findings of peripheral neuropathy secondary to ddI in phase I studies, no differences were found among the study arms. Despite prior expectations, no relation between duration of earlier zidovudine therapy and relative risk of clinical events favoring ddI was observed. Both doses of ddI produced small but significant increases in CD4 cell counts, compared with the zidovudine arm.

This study indicates the clinical activity of ddI in patients with low CD4 counts (without diagnosed AIDS) who had a median of 13.9 months of prior therapy with zidovudine. It is hoped that other ongoing studies will provide much-needed information for determining the optimal time to switch from zidovudine to ddI, and which patient population would benefit most. Another critical study (ACTG 116) compares zidovudine to ddI in patients with no prior antiretroviral therapy, and it should yield important information concerning optimal initial antiretroviral therapy.

In vitro evidence of resistance to ddI has developed in a small number of patients after approximately one year of therapy. It is usually the result of a single amino acid change in HIV-1 reverse transcriptase in the presence of at least one other amino acid change associated with decreased susceptibility to zidovudine. There have been small studies associating ddI susceptibility with CD4 and virologic changes but, as with zidovudine, the clinical significance of decreased in vitro susceptibility remains unclear.

ddC. As reported by Thomas C. Merigan and co-workers (ACTG protocol 012), low doses of ddC (0.01 mg/kg every eight hours or 0.005

mg/kg every four hours) have been effective in suppressing p24 antigen levels in patients with AIDS or advanced AIDS-related complex. Low doses do not enhance CD4 counts in patients with AIDS, but higher doses do produce increases in patients with ARC who can tolerate the therapy.

Hematologic toxicity is minimal with ddC. The principal toxicity is peripheral sensory neuropathy, which is dose dependent, cumulative, and can be severe, but is generally reversible, particularly when recognized early. Other side effects—stomatitis, rash, fever, and arthritis/arthralgia—are not dose dependent and are relatively uncommon. ACTG protocol 012 found that some patients tolerate extended low-dose ddC therapy without adverse effects and that there is a finite period during which neurotoxicity and other side effects are manifested. Neurotoxicity apparently develops during the first 24 weeks of therapy, whereas dermatologic changes most commonly occur during the first four to six weeks.

A large randomized trial of zidovudine versus ddC in AIDS/ARC patients who had had three months or less of prior zidovudine therapy was prematurely terminated in December 1991 because of a significantly higher death rate in the ddC arm as compared with the zidovudine arm. There were 320 patients on ddC and 315 on zidovudine; only 17% of the patients in either arm had ever received prior zidovudine therapy. The ddC arm was significantly inferior to zidovudine with respect to survival, occurrence of opportunistic infections or neoplasms, maximal CD4 cell increases, and the amount of time the CD4 count remained above baseline. Approximately 30% of all patients on ddC had developed moderate or severe neuropathy within the first year.

The FDA Advisory Committee on Antivirals did not recommend an indication for use of ddC monotherapy in April 1992. Whether ddC will have a role as monotherapy will have to await the conclusion of current ongoing trials being conducted by the ACTG and CPCRA. (The possible role of ddC in combination with zidovudine is discussed further on.) Resistance to ddC has been described in a small number of patients who had received therapy. It is associated with a single codon change in the reverse transcriptase gene. As with zidovudine and ddI administered in combination, the clinical significance remains uncertain.

D4T. The in vitro antiviral activity of D4T is similar to that of zidovudine, but its toxicity to bone marrow is substantially lower. In a phase I study (protocol 089), peripheral neuropathy and hepatic dysfunction were the dose-limiting toxicities. At doses that appear to be well tolerated, D4T has a positive effect on CD4 counts and p24 antigen. It is acid-stable and 100% bioavailable, and therefore it presents no difficulties in formulation or route of administration. A phase II comparative trial of ddI versus D4T is currently enrolling patients with AIDS.

AZdU. Like zidovudine, ddC, and D4T, AZdU is a pyrimidine nucleoside analogue. In Larder's study of zidovudine resistance, AZdU was the only antiretroviral agent to which cross-resistance was found. In comparison with zidovudine, a greater concentration of AZdU triphosphate is required to inhibit viral reverse transcriptase, but an even greater concentration is required to inhibit cellular DNA polymerases, so AZdU may be less toxic. In vitro evaluation in bone marrow cells suggests that AZdU may be substantially less myelosuppressive than zidovudine, but AZdU also has consistently less in vitro antiviral activity. AZdU is now in phase I studies.

3TC. 2'-deoxy-3'-thiacytidine is an analogue of deoxycytidine, in which a sulfur has replaced the COH group at the 3' position of the deoxyribose ring. The original racemic mixture (BCH-189) has now been separated with the (–) enantiomer (3TC) having the greater therapeutic index in cell lines. A phase I study is currently under way to evaluate clinical activity. This compound is a good example of how two closely related compounds could differ significantly in their in vitro toxicity.

Non-nucleoside reverse transcriptase inhibitors. A number of structurally unrelated compounds have been shown to specifically and potently inhibit HIV-1, but not HIV-2 or SIV reverse transcriptase. These compounds (TIBO, L697661, BIRG-587, U-87201E) were relatively nontoxic, but in clinical trials rapid emergence of resistance was found, with limited duration of antiviral activity. The development of in vivo resistance has been observed within eight weeks, both with and without concomitant zidovudine, in the clinical studies of L697661 and BIRG-587. This greater than 100-fold decrease in susceptibility of the virus is generally the result of one to two amino acid changes in the HIV-1 reverse transcriptase gene. Two agents of this class are currently under study at higher doses (BIRG-587 and U-87201E) to see if resistance of the virus can be overcome by higher concentrations of the drug.

Inhibitors of attachment. Binding to host cells occurs when the HIV envelope glycoprotein (gp120) binds to the CD4 receptor on the surface of the T lymphocyte. Inhibition of that process has been attempted with soluble CD4, a recombinant product of the extracellular portion of the receptor. In vitro, the soluble, truncated portion of the CD4 receptor binds to the HIV envelope glycoprotein and neutralizes its infectivity. Theoretically, therefore, soluble CD4 could prevent attachment of HIV to cells.

The logic behind the use of soluble CD4 is appealing (Figure 6), and an escalating dosage trial found no significant clinical or immunologic toxicity. Unfortunately, despite prolonged study and use of fairly high amounts of the agent, researchers have yet to establish a dose that has any apparent efficacy in terms of increasing CD4 counts or decreasing serum levels of viral p24 antigen. Recent data suggest a possible explanation: Binding of the soluble CD4 molecule to clinical isolates of HIV is

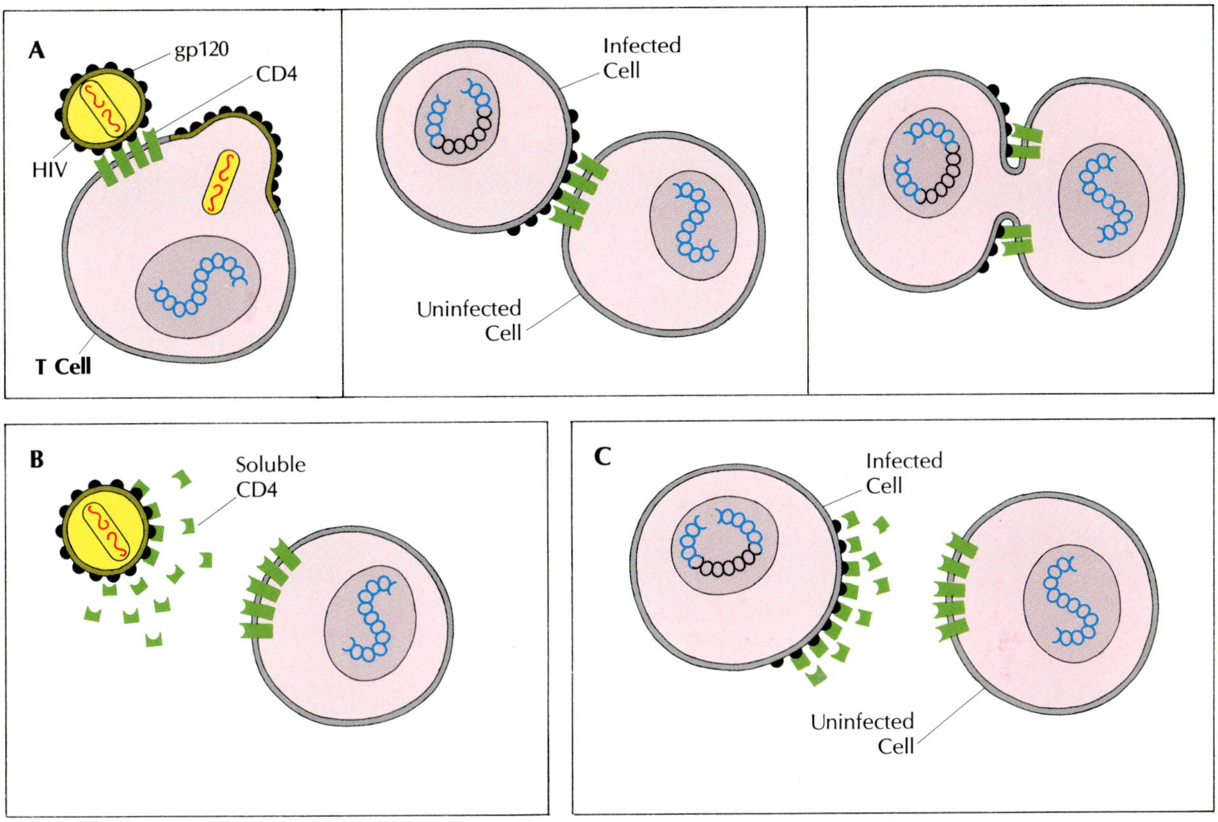

Figure 6 For HIV to infect a host cell, the virus must first attach to the cell membrane (A), an event believed to involve binding of viral gp120 ligands to CD4 receptors on T lymphocytes and other cells. Once infected, a cell expressing processed gp120 on its surface may fuse to another CD4-bearing host cell, forming a multinucleated giant cell. In theory, a soluble version of CD4 might prevent both viral attachment (B) and cell-to-cell spread (C).

much weaker than to the laboratory HIV strains originally tested. No further clinical trials are planned at this time.

Second-generation approaches to therapy involving CD4 are also under study. These include extending the half-life of CD4 by construction of a hybrid IgG molecule whose antigen-binding (Fc) region is replaced by the gp120-binding region of CD4 and by the construction of a chimeric molecule with a toxin. The binding of a high-affinity Fc receptor by the IgG CD4 suggests that mechanisms of pathogen elimination, such as phagocytosis and antibody-dependent cellular cytotoxicity, may be recruited to kill infected cells and virus. Early reports from the phase I trials of this hybrid molecule confirm that prolonged half-life has been achieved. Chimeric molecules—e.g., those with a CD4 binding domain linked to a toxin such as Pseudomonas exotoxin—are another variation using the specific gp120-CD4 binding approach. This molecule binds and is internalized, killing gp120-expressing cells. Early phase I studies have, however, been marked by toxicity, which may limit their usefulness.

An entirely new class of compounds, the glycosidase inhibitors, may also reduce HIV infectivity. In vitro, glycosidase inhibitors can reduce virus infectivity to varying degrees and prevent syncytia formation by inhibiting the cell's glycosylation pathways; however, these pathways are used by all cellular glycoproteins. The inability of these agents to specifically inhibit viral glycoprotein glycosylation has been the major impediment to progress in this area.

Inhibitors of viral protease. HIV protease is required for proper cleavage of the precursor HIV *gag* gene polyprotein into the correct functional structural proteins. Several candidate compounds have been developed that, in vitro, demonstrate specific inhibition of HIV-1 protease cleavage of the polyprotein—a step that is required for viral infectivity. A common difficulty with compounds in this class is that the requirements of the specific interactions for binding inhibition result in a large, poorly soluble molecule, which makes it difficult to produce an oral formulation with adequate bioavailability. It is expected that phase I trials of at least a few of the candidate compounds will begin within the year.

***tat* inhibitors.** The HIV-1 regulatory protein *tat* is required for HIV-1 transcription and viral replication. An inhibitor should therefore markedly decrease the formation of new viral RNA. One agent, Ro 24-7429, has so far been identified as a clinical candidate. Both *tat* and protease inhibitors have potential advantages, since they could affect chronically infected, virus-producing cells, which are not susceptible to the current reverse transcriptase inhibitors. Clinical trials of both classes of compounds are expected to begin shortly.

Combination therapy. Therapy with combinations of antiviral compounds has several theoretical advantages: It may reduce toxicity by permitting lower doses of active drugs; it may be more effective because of synergism (perhaps by attacking the virus at different stages of the replication process); and it may potentially reduce the opportunity for resistance. Potential drawbacks are increased toxicity, cost, complexity, and decreased compliance. Numerous combination studies are in progress or planned. The experience from other infectious diseases and oncology would indicate that the most effective combinations are those with agents having different mechanisms of action and toxicities.

Combinations of antiretroviral drugs and immunomodulators may have both a complementary and a synergistic effect in eradicating the virus from infected patients. Investigation of a possible synergistic effect of low-dose zidovudine or ddI and α2-interferon in patients with symptomatic HIV infection is now under way. An ACTG trial (protocol 024) has produced evidence of transient immunologic enhancement in asymptomatic patients treated with zidovudine plus continuous five-day infusions of interleukin-2 via an indwelling central venous catheter. The investigators are currently testing intermittent peripheral infusions of a new, long-acting form of interleukin-2 in conjunction with oral zidovudine.

Several small studies of concomitant or alternating therapy with zidovudine and ddC in patients without prior antiretroviral therapy have suggested that the duration of therapy-induced CD4 count elevation over baseline could be increased. Antiviral activity was similar to zidovudine alone, as would be expected, since it was used at a known active dose. Whether this will translate clinically into differences in disease progression and/or survival is the objective of several large randomized NIAID-sponsored trials. In contrast to their decision on ddC use as monotherapy, the FDA Advisory Committee on Antivirals recommended "accelerated" approval of concomitant zidovudine and ddC in patients with CD4 counts under 300 pending completion of the ongoing trials. The FDA has agreed, and the combination is currently licensed for adult patients with CD4 counts under 300 who have demonstrated significant clinical or immunologic deterioration after zidovudine therapy.

Immunomodulatory Therapies

Several proposed immunomodulatory therapies—including interferons, vaccination, thymic hormones, dimepranol acedoben with inosine, and ampligen—have been evaluated as monotherapies in HIV infection. For most of these agents, the data from well-controlled studies have been either nonsupportive or conflicting. However, the data have been promising for two classes of agents, interferons and vaccines, and they are under active investigation.

Interferons. The interferons are a large group of related cytokines in three families. The α-interferons have been the most widely studied. The use of α-interferon is an FDA-approved indication for therapy for Kaposi sarcoma, which is limited by the toxicity of high-dose therapy (flu-like syndrome, neutropenia, anemia, and hepatitis). In a randomized double-blind placebo-controlled trial conducted by the Interferon Alpha Study Group, administration of 3 million or 36 million units three times a week in 67 patients with AIDS demonstrated no significant effects on CD4 counts, p24 antigen levels, survival, or opportunistic infections. A randomized placebo-controlled trial has been conducted in 34 asymptomatic HIV-positive patients (CD4 counts greater than 400), using an average daily dose of 17.5 million units of α-interferon. The withdrawal and toxicity rates were high, but there was antiviral activity as demonstrated by a lower rate of HIV culture positivity and progression to AIDS. The CD4 percentage increased, but the CD4 number decreased compared with placebo.

Current trials are evaluating α-interferon in combination with zidovudine or ddI in patients with CD4 counts of 200 to 600. The combination of zidovudine and α-interferon is, however, limited by the additive bone marrow toxicity. Low-dose oral interferon was reported in an uncontrolled trial by Davy K. Koech and co-workers to induce HIV seroreversion, substantial increase in CD4 counts, and dramatic alleviation of clinical symptoms. However, no subsequent controlled trial has been able to confirm these findings. After reviewing the available data, an NIH advisory committee did not find evidence to support its use outside of the ongoing controlled trials.

Vaccines. The therapeutic use of vaccination to modify an infection has been examined since the latter part of the nineteenth century. Of the many different approaches investigated, two have stood the test of time and are currently in wide use: postexposure rabies vaccination and post-delivery hepatitis B vaccination. Unlike these viral illnesses, however, HIV infection progresses despite the development of specific antibody and cell-mediated immune responses. During the course of infection, the mutation of virus envelope occurs at a rate higher than that of influenza A, direct cell fusion can occur, and replication can occur in immunologically privileged sites—all of which may contribute to the host's apparent inability to contain the infection.

Many HIV vaccine candidates are under evaluation, based on recombinant envelope (gp160, gp120, or gp41), structural proteins (p24 or p17), and whole and subunit virions. Questions regarding adjuvants, source of viral strain, schedule and dose, and comparative immunity remain under active investigation. The largest body of clinical data has been elicited with a gp160 recombinant vaccine, which has been evaluated in small phase I studies in both normal volunteers and in HIV-infected patients. In both groups the vaccine appeared to be safe, with evidence of immune response that lasted approximately three months.

In HIV-infected patients, new humoral and cellular proliferative responses were observed. These were associated with CD4 counts greater than 600 at baseline (81% versus 43%) and the number of vaccinations received (87% for six versus 40% for three). There was some suggestion of CD4 stabilization in the vaccine responders, compared with a historical cohort. It is not known whether response to vaccine will translate into clinical benefit. Larger phase I/II trials and comparative phase II trials of different vaccine preparations are under active investigation.

Ineffective Agents

Studies by the ACTG and others have shown lack of efficacy of several drugs widely used by patients.

Ribavirin. Although ribavirin was claimed to have clinical utility in HIV infection, many small nonblinded trials in the mid-1980s failed to provide convincing evidence.The recently completed Spanish Ribavirin Trial, a large randomized double-blind study, demonstrated CD4 counts to be significantly lower with ribavirin than with placebo, and there was no evidence of antiviral or clinical activity. This was in agreement with earlier studies.

Dextran sulfate. This synthetic heparin analogue has anti-HIV activity in vitro, inhibiting both viral adsorption by cells and the formation of syncytia. It was widely used by patients in the late 1980s. An in vivo study (protocol 078) by Kevin J. Lorentsen and colleagues at Johns Hopkins demonstrated, however, that dextran sulfate is very poorly absorbed after oral administration. A later study showed that the drug had no antiviral activity when given parenterally, despite the development of full therapeutic anticoagulant activity. In addition, a significant incidence of thrombocytopenia was observed.

AL 721. Also widely used by patients at one time, this combination of fats purportedly derived its benefit from the 7 : 2 : 1 ratio of its three components. Studies of AL 721, however, demonstrated no positive effect on p24 antigen or CD4 counts, even at doses higher than those ordinarily used.

Zidovudine has proved to be an important palliative agent in all stages of HIV infection, enhancing both quality and length of life. ddI has been shown to be of clinical benefit in those who have previously been treated with zidovudine. Recently, the combination of zidovudine and ddC has been approved on the basis of surrogate marker activity. Its exact clinical role awaits the completion of ongoing trials. Many other anti-HIV agents are now under study and should begin to enter clinical use within a few years. Ultimately, therapeutic regimens in HIV infection may include a combination of these prospective agents, with or without zidovudine. Our long-range goals are, at the least, to render HIV infection a chronic, controllable disease and, at most, to eradicate it in those who have been infected.

SELECTED READING

Stein DS, Korvick JA, Vermund SH: CD4+ lymphocyte cell enumeration for prediction of clinical course of human immunodeficiency disease: A review. J Infect Dis 165 : 352, 1992

Lagakos S et al: Effects of zidovudine therapy in minority and other subpopulations with early HIV infection. JAMA 266 : 2709, 1991

Redfield RR et al: A phase I evaluation of the safety and immunogenicity of vaccination with recombinant gp160 in patients with early human immunodeficiency virus infection. N Engl J Med 324 : 1677, 1991

Graham NMH et al: The effects on survival of early treatment of human immunodeficiency virus infection. N Engl J Med 326 : 1037, 1992

Moore RD et al: Zidovudine and the natural history of the acquired immune deficiency syndrome. N Engl J Med 324 : 1412, 1991

Fischl MA et al: Prolonged zidovudine therapy in patients with AIDS and advanced AIDS-related complex. JAMA 262 : 2405, 1989

Schmitt FA et al: Neuropsychological outcome of zidovudine (AZT) treatment of patients with AIDS and AIDS-related complex. N Engl J Med 319:1573, 1988

Volberding PA et al: Zidovudine in asymptomatic human immunodeficiency virus infection. N Engl J Med 322:941, 1990

Fischl MA et al: The safety and efficacy of zidovudine (AZT) in the treatment of subjects with mildly symptomatic human immunodeficiency virus type 1 (HIV) infection. Ann Intern Med 112:727, 1990

Larder BA, Darby G, Richmann DD: HIV with reduced sensitivity to zidovudine (AZT) isolated during prolonged therapy. Science 243:1731, 1989

National Institute of Allergy and Infectious Diseases: AZT therapy for early HIV infection. Clinical Courier, vol 8, No. 5, 1990

5 Current Status of HIV Therapy: II. Opportunistic Diseases

JUDITH FEINBERG *and* DANIEL F. HOTH, JR.
Johns Hopkins University and *National Institute of Allergy and Infectious Diseases*

Acquired immune deficiency syndrome is characterized by infection with a wide variety of viruses, bacteria, fungi, and parasites and by the occurrence of certain malignancies. About 90% of deaths in patients infected with human immunodeficiency virus are directly or indirectly attributable to such opportunistic diseases. Antiretroviral therapy prolongs survival in patients with AIDS, but it has not reversed HIV-induced immunosuppression. In that context, the management and prevention of opportunistic diseases promises to become an even more pressing problem (Figure 1).

Many of the opportunistic diseases in AIDS are familiar because they occur in other immunocompromised patients, and even in some immunocompetent persons. Management in such cases often differs from that for AIDS patients, however. Medically induced immunosuppression, as in transplant recipients or cancer patients, can sometimes be moderated while the infection is brought under control. Because such immunosuppression is usually temporary, recovery from infection is possible. In untreated AIDS, immunosuppression progresses inexorably, although it may be stabilized for a time with antiretroviral therapy. Thus, initial control of an opportunistic infection may be more difficult and often must be followed by lifelong maintenance therapy, since the infection is suppressed rather than eradicated. Opportunistic diseases in AIDS patients may also require a different therapeutic approach because of differing pathophysiology. For example, cytomegalovirus tends to cause pneumonia in transplant recipients but retinitis

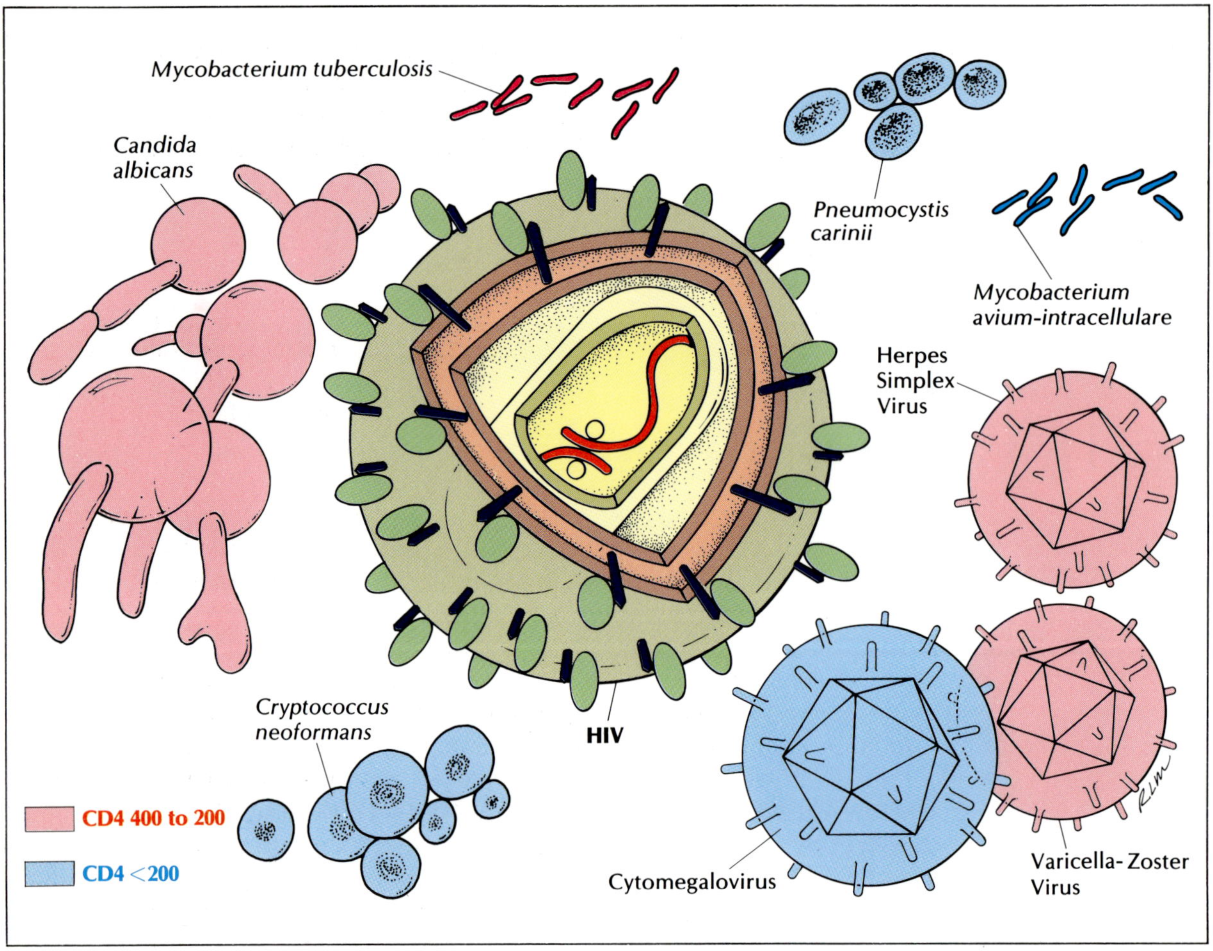

Figure 1 HIV infection follows a predictable course of progressive immunosuppression and increased susceptibility to certain infections and malignancies. In the context of the CD4 (helper T cell) count, the principal marker of HIV-induced immunosuppression, the infections tend also to occur in predictable patterns. When CD4 counts decline to about the 400 to 200 range, for example, zoster, herpes simplex, oropharyngeal candidiasis, and tuberculosis are common. Once counts drop below 200, the pathogenic possibilities broaden to include *Pneumocystis carinii*, *Cryptococcus neoformans*, cytomegalovirus, and *Mycobacterium avium-intracellulare*.

in AIDS patients. Finally, AIDS patients do not tolerate medications as well as other patients do, and they may have more severe or more frequent toxic reactions.

In the United States, much of the clinical research on opportunistic diseases is being carried out by the AIDS Clinical Trials Group (ACTG), which comprises investigators from 54 medical centers and operates under the auspices of the Division of AIDS of the NIAID. The ACTG's research strategy for opportunistic disease is multipronged. One goal is to test new agents or combinations in order to increase the number of therapeutic options available (this may include expanding the indications for agents currently marketed). Another is to replace agents that require frequent intravenous dosing with oral therapies or parenteral agents that have long half-lives. The strategy involves research on both the treatment of acute opportunistic infections and their prophylaxis. The ultimate goal is to prevent opportunistic illness by supplanting therapy with prophylaxis.

Pneumocystis carinii Pneumonia (PCP)

PCP is the most common opportunistic infection in advanced HIV disease. In the past, as many as 80% of AIDS patients had at least one episode of PCP; adoption of PCP prophylaxis may be reducing that percentage. PCP is one of the most commonly documented causes of death in AIDS. Among hospitalized AIDS patients, each episode of PCP results in 10% to 30% mortality.

Current standard therapies for PCP are co-trimoxazole (trimethoprim-sulfamethoxazole) and parenteral pentamidine. Both are effective, but for some reason AIDS patients are extremely vulnerable to side effects, with dose-limiting toxicity developing in 30% to 60%. The search for less toxic regimens, as well as for oral regimens for patients who are less severely ill, has produced a number of alternatives, some of which have gained wide use. One popular oral combination, which has not yet completed prospective comparison with other regimens, is dapsone and trimethoprim. Like sulfamethoxazole, dapsone inhibits dihydropteroate synthase (DHPS), an enzyme critical to microbial synthesis of folate. Trimethoprim inhibits the related enzyme dihydrofolate reductase (DHFR).

After it was observed that the antimalarial effect of primaquine was enhanced by mirincamycin (a lincosamine antibiotic similar to clindamycin), the combination of primaquine and clindamycin was investigated in PCP. Animal studies showed that although each agent alone had little or no effect, the combination of the two was extremely effective for both prophylaxis and treatment.

Preliminary results of a clinical trial of intravenous and oral clindamycin and oral primaquine in AIDS patients with mild to moderate PCP suggested a response rate of 90% or more, with toxicity requiring discontinuance of the drugs in 18%. This combination is gaining wide clinical use, although it has not yet been directly compared with standard therapy.

Aerosolized pentamidine has been used to avoid the toxicity seen with parenteral administration. One comparative study of aerosolized pentamidine found that mortality was slightly lower than with co-trimoxazole, but resolution of symptoms was slower. Aerosolized pentamidine should probably be limited to use in patients with mild to moderate disease, as drug deposition in the lungs is regional and optimal distribution is effort dependent.

The combination of trimetrexate and leucovorin calcium showed early promise for moderately severe PCP. Trimetrexate, a DHFR inhibitor, is significantly more potent in vitro than pyrimethamine and trimethoprim; leucovorin prevents trimetrexate's toxicity to mammalian cells, yet does not inhibit its antiprotozoal effect. Trimetrexate is given intravenously, leucovorin IV or orally. However, a controlled trial suggested that co-trimoxazole therapy was superior to trimetrexate. One possible reason for this is that trimetrexate inhibits only DHFR, whereas co-trimoxazole inhibits DHPS as well. Sequential blockade of these two essential enzymes in the folate pathway may be therapeutically crucial. However, trimetrexate is clearly active in PCP and might provide salvage therapy for patients intolerant of or unresponsive to standard therapies.

Another antimalarial, atovaquone, has proved useful for acute PCP. Despite the fact that it was the first agent to appear "cidal" in animal studies, it was less effective when compared with co-trimoxazole, although it was better tolerated. Its limited effectiveness is likely due to poor oral bioavailability.

Adjuvant steroid therapy. Many patients with PCP get worse before they get better, deteriorating for several days after initiation of treatment and then subsequently showing improvement. A possible cause of this phenomenon may be increased pulmonary inflammation, perhaps from accumulation of dead or dying organisms after specific therapy is initiated. In this context, systemic corticosteroids have been studied as adjuvant therapy in patients with PCP.

Recent results of a large randomized study suggest that steroids started within 36 hours of specific antiprotozoal therapy are effective in blunting the early deterioration in oxygenation and in enhancing survival. Best results were in moderately to severely ill patients (Figure 2). The number of mildly ill patients was too limited for an effect to be discernible.

These findings are supported by three small randomized studies that also initiated steroids early (within 72 hours of starting conventional therapy). Results of these studies are the basis for a consensus panel's recommendations on use of adjuvant steroids in moderate to severe PCP, defined as room air blood gases with a Pao_2 less than 70 torr or an (A-a) Do_2 greater than 35 torr. The panel recommended the modest doses used in the largest study: 40 mg of prednisone twice a day for five days, followed by 40 mg once a day for five days, and then 20 mg daily for 11 days.

Prophylaxis. Clinical research has shown that patients who have had one episode of PCP benefit greatly from prophylaxis against future episodes. Without secondary prophylaxis, at least 45% of patients who survive the first episode will have a second within two years.

Three hundred milligrams of aerosolized pentamidine, delivered by jet nebulizer once monthly, has been shown to lower that risk of recurrence to about 20% annually among symptomatic patients with advanced HIV disease. This regimen was more effective than 150 or 30 mg of

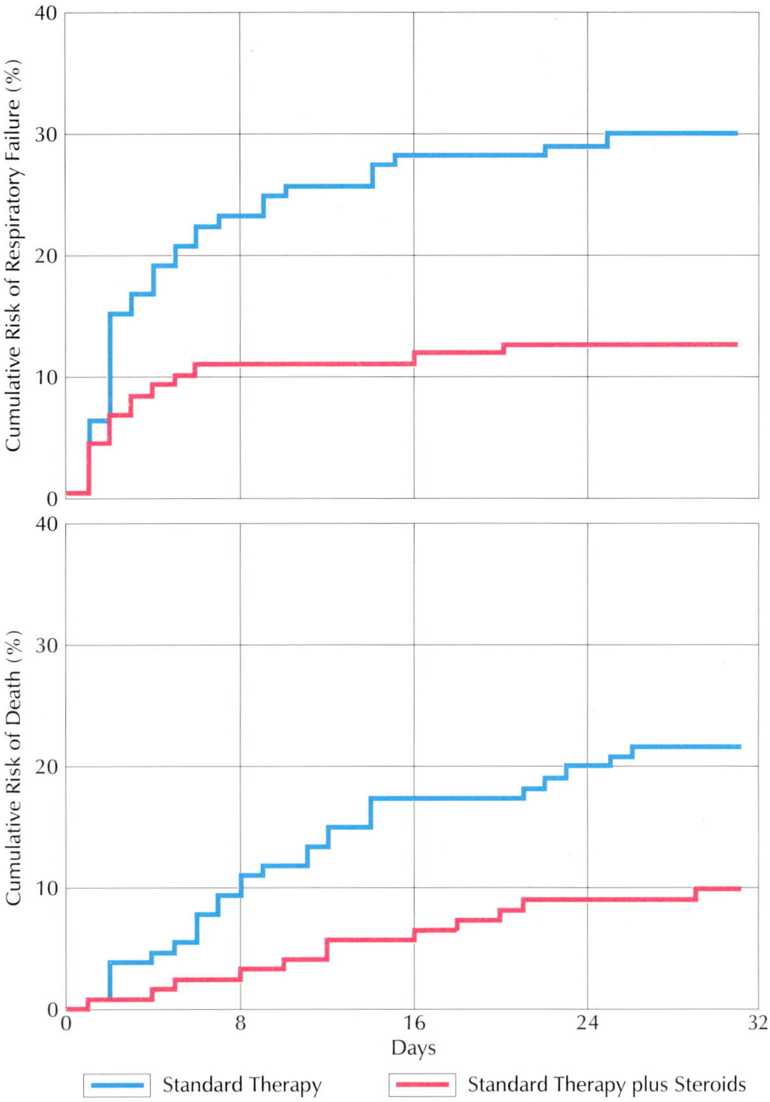

Figure 2 In a randomized trial by Samuel A. Bozzette and colleagues at the California Collaborative Treatment Group, 251 AIDS patients known or presumed to have *Pneumocystis carinii* pneumonia received standard therapy (co-trimoxazole, pentamidine, or dapsone and trimethoprim) with or without adjuvant corticosteroids. In steroid-treated patients, the cumulative risk of respiratory failure during an episode of pneumonia was significantly lowered (top), as was the cumulative risk of death (bottom).

the drug given every two weeks (Figure 3). Because of uneven regional deposition, however, breakthrough pneumonias may occur in patients on aerosolized pentamidine. Aerosolized pentamidine has also been used effectively with a different dose, 150 mg every two weeks, when delivered by a hand-held ultrasonic nebulizer. These breakthroughs often involve the upper lobe and may present as extensive apical cystic lesions. Other limitations of aerosolized pentamidine prophylaxis include its associa-

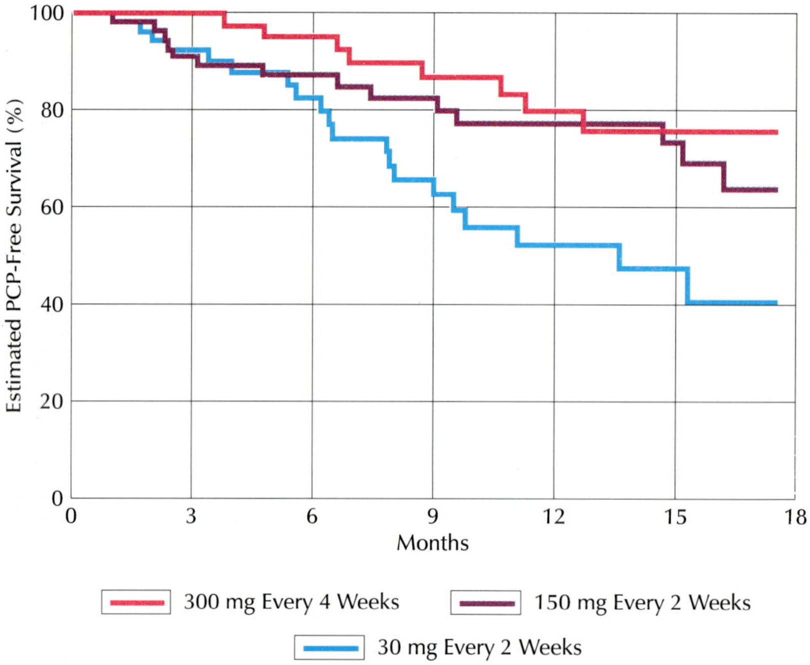

Figure 3 In a trial of aerosolized pentamidine for prevention of *Pneumocystis carinii* pneumonia, 208 patients who had had PCP were randomized to 300 mg of the drug every four weeks, or to 150 or 30 mg every two weeks. Comparison of estimated PCP-free survival in the three groups showed that the 300-mg regimen was significantly more effective than the 30-mg regimen. The trend of the data in this study also suggested a long-term advantage in the 300-mg group compared with the 150-mg group.

tion with the development of extrapulmonary pneumocystosis and its narrow spectrum of coverage (e.g., it does not protect against toxoplasmosis or bacterial infection).

Data from a prospective randomized trial of secondary prophylaxis comparing co-trimoxazole, one double-strength tablet daily, and aerosolized pentamidine, 300 mg monthly, have shown that there were significantly fewer recurrences among co-trimoxazole recipients. The estimated one-year recurrence rate was 18.5% for the aerosolized pentamidine group as compared with 3.5% for the co-trimoxazole group.

Dapsone also provides effective PCP prophylaxis according to numerous small or uncontrolled studies. A large study comparing dapsone, co-trimoxazole, and aerosolized pentamidine for primary prevention of PCP is ongoing.

It should be noted that the at-risk population for PCP has been defined by epidemiologic studies in the Multicenter AIDS Cohort Study (MACS). Recommendations by the U.S. Public Health Service to provide primary prophylaxis to individuals with total CD4 counts of less than 200 are based on the rate of PCP development among HIV-infected men (Figure 4).

On the basis of the results described above, the Public Health Service has recently revised its recommendations for PCP prophylaxis. Co-tri-

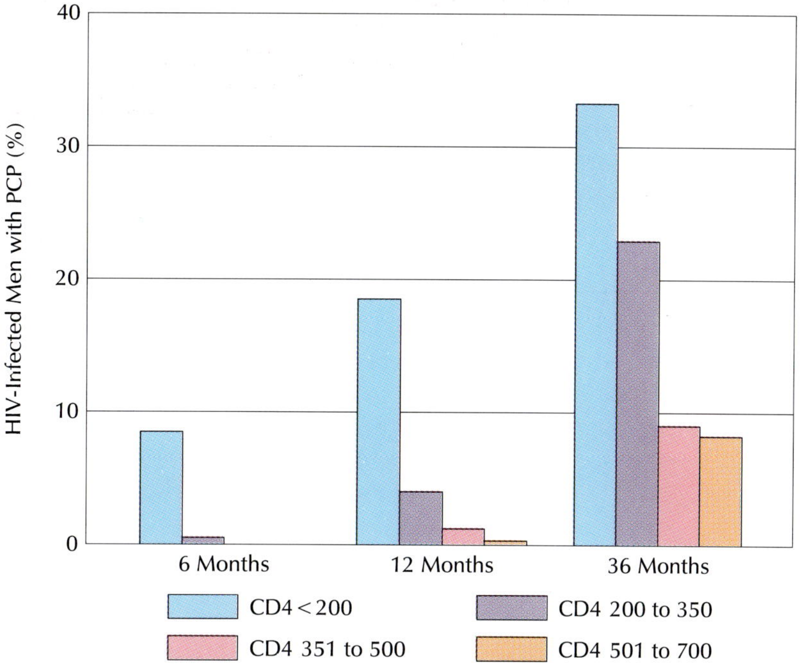

Figure 4 The Multicenter AIDS Cohort Study found that *Pneumocystis carinii* pneumonia (PCP) was most frequent in HIV-infected men with CD4 counts under 200. The rate rose from less than 10% in the six months after the first <200 count was obtained to more than 30% at 36 months. Among those whose CD4 depletion was not as severe, PCP was rare or nonexistent at six months and infrequent at 12 months. At 36 months, however, the pneumonia had occurred in more than 20% of men with initial CD4 counts of 200 to 350.

moxazole is now the preferred form of prophylaxis. For patients who cannot tolerate this agent, aerosolized pentamidine delivered by jet or ultrasonic nebulizer is an effective alternative.

Fungal Infections

Advanced HIV infection is often complicated by severe fungal infections, which may be life threatening. In endemic areas—and among patients with a history of residence or travel in those areas—mycoses such as histoplasmosis, blastomycosis, and coccidioidomycosis cause significant morbidity and mortality. In arid areas of the Southwest, for example, coccidioidomycosis is the third most common opportunistic infection in AIDS.

Although AIDS patients with systemic mycoses generally show a good clinical response to primary treatment with amphotericin B, the relapse rate 12 months after primary treatment is 90%, compared with 10% to 20% in non-AIDS patients. Earlier in the epidemic, oral ketoconazole had been used to prevent relapse in AIDS patients, but it was unsuccessful in up to 50%. Postulated reasons for those failures include poor absorption and lack of potency.

Oropharyngeal candidiasis is one of the earliest opportunistic diseases in HIV infection and is almost universal. It causes pain, dysphagia, and anorexia. Invasive fungal diseases occur later in the course of HIV disease when immunosuppression is severe. A study is under way to compare the efficacy of fluconazole versus clotrimazole in preventing serious fungal infection, including esophageal candidiasis and systemic mycoses, as well as limited mucocutaneous infection.

Histoplasmosis. Disseminated histoplasmosis is a life-threatening opportunistic infection in patients with AIDS. In endemic areas of the Midwest, the disease develops in 5% to 10% of AIDS patients. Outbreaks of pulmonary histoplasmosis among the general population, which have occurred in Indianapolis in recent years, can push the rate higher in a given locality. Histoplasmosis can occur by reactivation as well as by primary infection in patients with AIDS, hence the disease may recur years after an exposed person has left an endemic area.

The triazole compound itraconazole has been used successfully to treat disseminated histoplasmosis in non-AIDS patients. It has greater in vitro activity, is more predictably absorbed, and is better tolerated than ketoconazole. Oral itraconazole is now being studied for primary treatment and suppression of relapse in AIDS patients as well as for suppression of relapse after successful acute therapy with amphotericin B.

Cryptococcal infection. Cryptococcosis, most commonly meningitis but also pneumonitis or disseminated infection, has been reported in 2% to 13% of AIDS patients. Because the causative organism is ubiquitous, cryptococcal infections occur in AIDS patients in all regions of the United States.

Cryptococcal meningitis, along with toxoplasmosis, is among the most common CNS infections in AIDS patients. Standard therapy for acute cryptococcal meningitis—amphotericin B with or without flucytosine—is effective in HIV-infected patients. Relapse is common, however, and maintenance therapy is complicated by the toxicity of amphotericin B and the difficulties of long-term intravenous suppressive therapy.

Fluconazole, an oral triazole, was recently approved by the FDA for treatment of acute cryptococcal meningitis in AIDS. In a study comparing fluconazole with amphotericin B, overall mortality was almost 20% in both arms, although a larger proportion of fluconazole recipients died within the first 14 days—19 (15%) versus five (8%) on amphotericin B. Culture conversion occurred significantly earlier in amphotericin B–treated patients. Results of another study, however, have shown that, compared with weekly intravenous administration of 1 mg/kg of amphotericin B, oral fluconazole, 200 mg daily, is the drug of choice for long-term suppression following acute therapy. The inadequate response of AIDS patients to standard therapy with amphotericin B has led to renewed enthusiasm for the combination of amphotericin and flucytosine. A prospective randomized study to assess the potential benefit of flucytosine is currently ongoing.

Toxoplasmosis

Typically, toxoplasmosis in HIV-infected patients occurs by reactivation rather than de novo acquisition. The usual site of infection is the brain. Toxoplasmosis has a geographic association, although not as clearly defined as that for endemic mycoses such as histoplasmosis. In general, the warmer the climate, the greater the prevalence. In the Western Hemisphere, the disease is much more common in the Caribbean than in the northern United States. Hence, the disease is seen much more frequently in areas with large concentrations of Caribbean immigrants, such as Miami and New York City.

Standard therapy for toxoplasmic encephalitis—pyrimethamine and sulfadiazine—is often not well tolerated by AIDS patients. Clindamycin plus pyrimethamine is a commonly used alternative regimen. Several promising new drugs such as azithromycin, clarithromycin, and atovaquone are being tested currently. There are also ongoing studies of pyrimethamine for prophylaxis of toxoplasmosis. Co-trimoxazole may confer a protective benefit against toxoplasmosis as well as PCP.

Herpesvirus Infections

Severe and prolonged mucocutaneous herpesvirus infection has been reported in AIDS patients, and serologic studies show a high prevalence of HSV infection in HIV-infected men. HSV infection in immunocompetent hosts is treated with acyclovir. With prolonged and repeated use, in vitro resistance to acyclovir may occur, and clinical resistance to the drug is an emerging problem in AIDS patients.

In most cases, the mechanism of HSV resistance to acyclovir is markedly diminished activity of virus-specified thymidine kinase, which phosphorylates acyclovir and permits it to act as a competitive inhibitor of viral DNA polymerase. Consequently, almost all HSV strains that are resistant to acyclovir should remain susceptible to both vidarabine and foscarnet (trisodium phosphonoformate), since vidarabine is phosphorylated entirely by cellular enzymes and foscarnet does not require phosphorylation for activity. However, a randomized comparison of foscarnet and vidarabine for acyclovir-resistant mucocutaneous HSV infection in AIDS patients showed foscarnet to be both better tolerated and more effective. Topical therapy with trifluridine, marketed for the treatment of herpes keratitis, is being studied. Preliminary results are encouraging, and there has been no systemic toxicity to date.

Cytomegalovirus

In the general population, infection with cytomegalovirus is common and generally benign. Beyond the perinatal period, CMV usually causes subclinical illness or at most a transient syndrome resembling mononucleosis. Thereafter, it remains in the body but is kept in check by the immune system. Among persons with AIDS, CMV causes considerable morbidity and mortality. At autopsy, evidence of CMV infection in the retina, gastrointestinal tract, lungs, liver, and central nervous system is found in more than 90% of AIDS patients.

Retinitis. The most common manifestation of disseminated CMV infection in persons with AIDS is retinitis. CMV retinitis is estimated to affect approximately 20% of AIDS patients. The virus reaches the retina via hematogenous dissemination and causes irreversible retinal necrosis. Without treatment, lesions progressively enlarge, causing visual field defects and, ultimately, blindness. CMV retinitis signifies profound immunocompromise—median CD4 lymphocyte counts in these patients are typically less than 50. The ultimate prognosis for both vision and survival is poor; survival after diagnosis was initially described as less than four months.

Both ganciclovir and foscarnet have been approved by the FDA for treatment of CMV retinitis. Initial response ranges from approximately 80% to 100%, with remission rates estimated at 60% and 80%. Figure 5 shows time to first progression of CMV retinitis in patients treated with ganciclovir through a treatment IND program that provided access to the drug prior to its licensure. A recently completed study compared the two drugs. Both were equally effective in controlling CMV retinitis. Although foscarnet was more toxic than ganciclovir, patients randomized to foscarnet had survival extended by four months. This was not fully explained but may be due to foscarnet's intrinsic anti-HIV activity, its synergistic effect against HIV when used with zidovudine, and/or its lack of myelosuppression, which permits concurrent use of recommended doses of zidovudine.

The optimal timing for initiating ganciclovir treatment for HIV-infected patients with CMV retinitis has not been established. Prompt treatment is generally advised for posterior-pole retinitis, which poses an immediate threat to vision, but deferred treatment is sometimes recommended for disease confined to the peripheral retina. Deferring treatment until lesions become posterior reduces the risk of drug-related toxicity, primarily neutropenia for ganciclovir and renal dysfunction for foscarnet. Resistant CMV isolates have been reported after therapy with both agents. Combined therapy is being explored as an avenue to increased effectiveness and to delayed emergence of resistance.

At present, intravenous therapy with either agent is used in a two-step approach. After two to three weeks of intensive induction therapy, lifelong lower-dose maintenance therapy is given to prevent progression or reactivation of retinitis. Maintenance therapy requires long-term intravenous access, such as a Hickman catheter. Ganciclovir-induced neutropenia can be sufficiently severe to require temporary withdrawal of the drug; the neutrophil count subsequently recovers, but repeated interruption of therapy may result in relapse of retinitis. The addition of a neutrophil-stimulating cytokine, such as granulocyte colony-stimulating

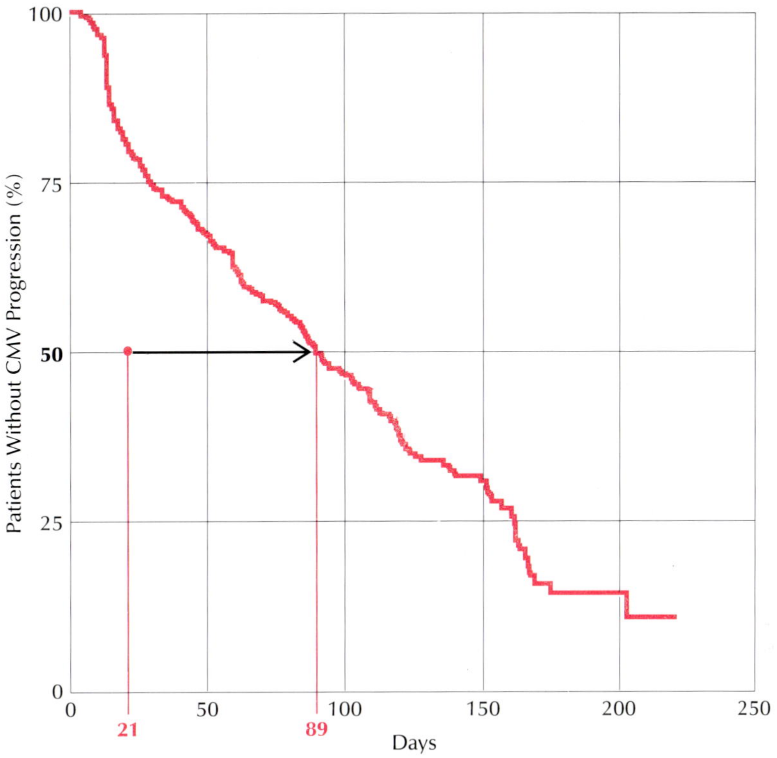

Figure 5 Results in 701 patients suggest that ganciclovir therapy may slow the progression of cytomegalovirus retinitis, which develops in profoundly immunosuppressed AIDS patients and is difficult to treat. Although the proportion of those patients in whom newly diagnosed CMV retinitis did not progress steadily declined, the median time that passed before the first evidence of the disease's progression was 89 days. In contrast, the median time to progression of CMV retinitis in the absence of maintenance therapy has been reported to be on the order of 21 days. Thus, therapy was associated with a large shift to the right with respect to the time course of progression (arrow at 50% level).

factor or granulocyte-macrophage colony-stimulating factor, has been used to prevent or to ameliorate neutropenia. Renal insufficiency due to foscarnet is managed by dose reduction or interruption. Hydration with intravenous saline has been effective in minimizing nephrotoxicity.

As an alternative to systemic administration (with its consequent risk of myelosuppression), ganciclovir can be injected directly into the affected eye. Anecdotal reports have shown good results with the technique.

Foscarnet also has a role as salvage therapy for CMV retinitis in patients intolerant of or unable to take ganciclovir because of baseline myelosuppression or ganciclovir resistance. Unfortunately, patients with CMV retinitis are generally sicker than those with HSV infection, require higher doses of foscarnet—90 or 120 mg/kg a day, compared with 40 mg/kg a day for resistant HSV—and do not tolerate the drug as well.

Reversible impairment in renal function can occur, necessitating dose adjustment. Neurotoxicity has occurred at doses of 120 mg/kg a day. Several patients have had symptomatic hypocalcemia during or immediately after infusion due to chelation by the drug. Because of potential cation shifts, foscarnet must be administered by an infusion pump over one to two hours.

Oral agents. An effective oral drug for maintenance therapy would avoid lifelong placement of an indwelling central venous catheter, as is required with both ganciclovir and foscarnet, and could be explored as preventive therapy. Current possibilities are oral ganciclovir and the acyclovir prodrug BW256U87, both of which are being tested currently as prophylaxis and, in the case of oral ganciclovir, for maintenance therapy of retinitis.

Mycobacterial Infection

Tuberculosis is a very aggressive disease in HIV-infected persons. It may develop when CD4 lymphocyte counts are still above 400. Fortunately, HIV-infected persons infected with sensitive strains of tuberculosis respond to standard therapy. However, the recent emergence of multidrug-resistant TB on the East Coast—primarily in New York and Miami—presents a clinical and public health problem with enormous potential impact. Therapeutic options are limited for multidrug-resistant tuberculosis, as some isolates have been resistant to all first-line drugs and many second- and third-line agents as well. In contrast, infection with *Mycobacterium avium-intracellulare* (MAI)—or *M. avium* complex, as it is also known—tends to be an end-stage occurrence. MAI is ubiquitous in soil and water and has very low pathogenicity; in fact, for some time there was debate over whether it was a commensal.

MAI infection is difficult to treat because of its resistance to most antituberculosis drugs. In tuberculosis, use of combination therapy prevents emergence of resistance; in MAI infection, multiple drugs are necessary to overcome intrinsic resistance and to produce even a modest therapeutic effect.

Whether chemotherapy for MAI may be effective in reducing mortality is currently unknown. Uncontrolled studies have evaluated single agents, of which the most active is ethambutol, as well as multidrug regimens that include ciprofloxacin, ethambutol, rifampin, clofazimine, and parenteral amikacin. In these studies, quantitative blood cultures and systemic symptoms (fever, night sweats, weight gain, diarrhea) have been assessed. More recently, the newer macrolides, azithromycin and clarithromycin, have been evaluated as single-drug therapy for MAI bacteremia. In these studies as in the earlier ones, blood culture yields decreased, and there was some improvement in systemic symptoms. No information on prolonged therapy has been obtained. Development of tolerable and effective regimens for MAI infections in AIDS patients is a high priority for current research.

Oncology

Kaposi sarcoma. This is often a relatively early manifestation of AIDS, occurring when immune competence is more or less intact, and it appears to be for the most part confined to homosexual and bisexual men. Over the course of the AIDS epidemic, it has become somewhat less common.

Kaposi sarcoma has two basic manifestations, mucocutaneous and visceral. Mucocutaneous lesions can be monitored and treatment initiated when discomfort or concern about appearance warrants intervention. Many approaches—including local irradiation, α-interferon, oral VP-16 (etoposide), vincristine, and vinblastine—have been used to manage this form of the disease with reasonable success.

Kaposi sarcoma that disseminates to visceral organs is debilitating and can be fatal; pulmonary KS is especially aggressive. Combination chemotherapy is the standard approach, and success has been limited. The choice of agents tends to vary with regional preference, but one popular combination is ABV: doxorubicin (Adriamycin), bleomycin, and vincristine or vinblastine. Angiogenesis inhibitors offer future promise as therapeutic agents as they are directed against the pathogenesis of Kaposi sarcoma.

Non-Hodgkin's lymphoma. As long as the root problem in HIV-induced immunosuppression remains unsolved, reduction of one opportunistic disease may simply clear the way for another. There are early suggestions that as Pneumocystis pneumonia becomes less common with more successful prophylaxis and therapy, lymphoma may be taking its place. Long-term follow-up in a limited number of AIDS patients on antiretroviral therapy has shown lymphoma rates to be as high as 15%.

Lymphoma has an established history as an opportunisitic malignancy in transplant recipients and other immunosuppressed patients, and conventional regimens are effective in HIV-infected patients. Patients with HIV are, however, much more vulnerable to the side effects of those regimens, particularly bone marrow suppression. Patients with AIDS tend to have fragile bone marrow reserves in any case, because of the HIV infection itself, zidovudine therapy, and other opportunistic infections that affect the bone marrow.

The first protocol to be adapted for HIV-related lymphoma was mBACOD: methotrexate, bleomycin, doxorubicin, cyclophosphamide, vincristine (Oncovin), and dexamethasone. Reduced doses of mBACOD have produced reasonably good responses. The addition of GM-CSF to improve tolerance to mBACOD is now being studied.

Primary CNS lymphoma is becoming more common in AIDS. CNS lymphomas are particularly aggressive and hard to treat in AIDS patients. Regrettably, no significant advances in therapy have yet been made.

HIV-infected patients should be monitored closely so that any opportunistic illness can be detected early in its course. Prompt control of acute infection and sustained suppression thereafter are critical for survival. Ultimately, as appropriate broad-spectrum agents are developed, it is anticipated that multiple opportunistic pathogen prophylaxis can be provided by a limited number of drugs.

SELECTED READING

Mills J, Masur H: AIDS-related infections. Sci Am 263(2):50, 1990

Feinberg J, Mills J: Treatment of opportunistic infections. AIDS 4(suppl 1): S209, 1991

Feinberg J et al: Update on opportunistic infections AIDS 5(suppl 2): S195, 1992

Sattler FR, Feinberg J: New developments in the treatment of *Pneumocystic carinii* pneumonia. Chest 101:451, 1992

Crowe SM et al: Predictive value of CD4 lymphocyte numbers for the development of opportunistic infections and malignancies in HIV-infected persons. J AIDS 4:770, 1991

Feinberg J: OI update: Current clinical research. AIDS Clin Care 3:42, 1991

Studies of Ocular Complications of AIDS Research Group, AIDS Clinical Trials Group: Mortality in patients with the acquired immunodeficiency syndrome treated with either foscarnet or ganciclovir for cytomegalovirus retinitis. N Engl J Med 326:213, 1992

Kemper CA et al: Treatment of *Mycobacterium avium* complex bacteremia in AIDS with a four-drug oral regimen. Ann Intern Med 116:466, 1992

Esplin JA, Levine AM: HIV-related neoplastic disease: 1991. AIDS 5(suppl 2):S203, 1992

Powderly WG et al: A controlled trial of fluconazole or amphotericin B to prevent relapse of cryptococcal meningitis in patients with the acquired immunodeficiency syndrome. N Engl J Med 326:793, 1992

Saag MS et al: Comparison of amphotericin B with fluconazole in the treatment of acute AIDS-associated cryptococcal meningitis. N Engl J Med 326:83, 1992

Montaner JSG et al: Aerosol pentamidine for secondary prophylaxis of AIDS-related: A randomized, placebo-controlled study. Ann Intern Med 114: 948, 1991

Leoung GS et al: Aerosolized pentamidine for prophylaxis against *Pneumocystis carinii* pneumonia. N Engl J Med 323:769, 1990

Centers for Disease Control: Guidelines for prophylaxis against *Pneumocystis carinii* pneumonia for persons infected with human immunodeficiency virus. MMWR 41(RR4):1, 1992

Bozzette SA et al: Controlled trial of early adjunctive treatment with corticosteroids for *Pneumocystis carinii* pneumonia in the acquired immunodeficiency syndrome. N Engl J Med 323:1451, 1990

Masur H et al: Consensus statement of the use of corticosteroids as adjuctive therapy for Pneumocystis pneumonia in the acquired immunodeficiency syndrome. N Engl J Med 323:1500, 1990

6 The Prospects for AIDS Vaccines

WAYNE C. KOFF *National Institute of Allergy and Infectious Diseases*

Historically, vaccines are among the best measures for preventing and controlling disease. Ever since human immunodeficiency virus was identified as the cause of AIDS, the development of vaccines against HIV has been a high priority.

The obstacles involved are formidable: If viruses were ranked in terms of the difficulties they present to developers of vaccines, HIV would clearly be the gold standard. Nonetheless, recent studies have provided grounds for optimism that a safe and effective AIDS vaccine is feasible. Furthermore, AIDS vaccine research is spinning off technologic developments applicable to the production of vaccines against other viral diseases.

Efficacy Issues

Two critical questions in the development of an AIDS vaccine are what components of the immune system must be enlisted to protect against the virus (Figure 1), and what antigenic components of the virus must a vaccine contain to induce that protective response.

With vaccines against other viral illnesses, such as poliomyelitis, measles, and hepatitis, the achievement of immunity correlates with production of neutralizing antibodies against the virus. Correlates of immunity to HIV are only now beginning to emerge. Neutralizing antibodies in persons infected with HIV, for example, are generally at low titers and do not halt progression to AIDS.

Along with neutralizing antibodies, cell-mediated immune responses may be necessary to buttress protection against the virus. Antigenic stimulation of monocytes and T cells causes the release of cytokines that can activate natural killer cells and macrophages, which can then kill HIV-infected cells in vitro. Moreover, antibodies specific for HIV can arm killer

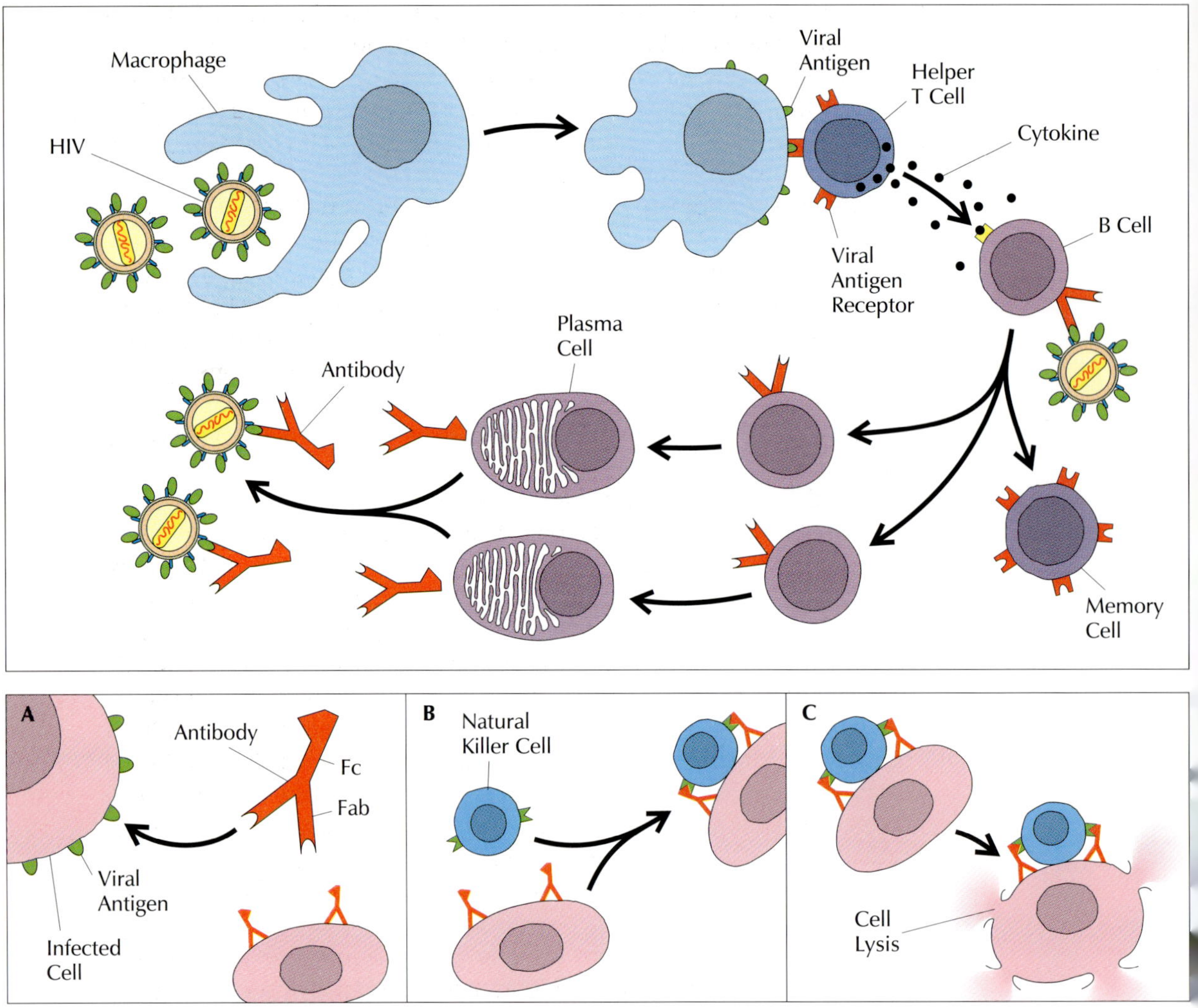

Figure 1 Successful vaccines against various viral diseases stimulate neutralizing antibody production. As in natural infection (top), this response involves macrophage presentation of viral antigen to helper CD4 cells, whose secretion of cytokines stimulates proliferation of B cells that have also encountered the antigen. The B cells then differentiate into specific antibody-secreting plasma cells and into specific memory cells capable of mounting an anamnestic response. Antibody-dependent cellular cytotoxicity (bottom) may also be relevant to viral vaccine efficacy. ADCC involves antibody coating of virally infected cells (A), natural killer cell binding to the Fc domain of the antibody (B), and lysis of infected cells (C). Cytotoxic CD8 cells, also capable of lysing virally infected cells (not shown), may be another critical component of vaccine-induced immune response.

cells to destroy virus-infected cells in the mechanism known as antibody-dependent cellular cytotoxicity (ADCC). As with other viruses that, like HIV, have an envelope, ADCC may be important in protecting against in vivo challenge.

A stumbling block in AIDS vaccine development has been the lack of a readily available animal model in which to test candidate vaccines. Chimpanzees are being used because they seroconvert and generate HIV-specific T-cell responses after inoculation with HIV, and the virus can subsequently be isolated from peripheral mononuclear cells. HIV infection does not, however, produce an AIDS-like disease in chimpanzees. Furthermore, the number of chimpanzees available for AIDS vaccine testing in the United States is limited.

Certain strains of simian immunodeficiency virus (SIV) produce an AIDS-like disease in rhesus macaques, with declining CD4 lymphocyte counts and death from opportunistic infection after an average of eight to 10 months. SIV differs from HIV in a number of respects, but the consensus is that the SIV model is as close a match for HIV as can be expected and the number of animals available for study is adequate. Consequently, vaccine developers are performing experiments in the SIV-macaque system with the expectation that a successful strategy would also work against HIV.

Several types of candidate vaccine have in fact been shown to protect against establishment of HIV or SIV infection in the chimpanzee or macaque model, respectively. That protection was demonstrated, however, in experiments designed to provide the best possible chance of a positive result. There are, in fact, four aspects of the experiments that deviate from conditions commonly found in nature: After vaccination and boosting, the study animals were challenged almost immediately—a week or two after the final immunization. In addition, they were challenged with a virus homologous to that used in the vaccine; they were challenged intravenously, rather than by mucosal exposure; and they were challenged with free rather than intracellular virus. The success of those studies made 1990 the first year in which some optimism about AIDS vaccines began to emerge; however, the limitations of the studies sound a cautionary note.

Studies to test the efficacy of vaccines under conditions that are less than ideal are now being planned or initiated. They will include challenge with heterologous isolates and infected cells, challenge by variable routes, and delayed challenge. Most will be in the SIV system. Since the goal is not to protect macaques against SIV infection but to protect humans against HIV infection, however, the safety and efficacy of prototype vaccines will have to be assessed in healthy, HIV-seronegative humans. Several such studies are in progress, and participating subjects have generated a range of humoral and cellular immune responses to candidate vaccines. When the lines of evidence from the monkey and human studies converge, which could be within a few years, we may be able to choose candidate vaccines for large-scale clinical trials.

Assembling that evidence will be a difficult and time-consuming task. The NIAID has established two closely integrated programs—the AIDS Vaccine Research and Development Group and the AIDS Vaccine Clinical Trials Network—to help bring vaccines from basic research to clinical testing. The institute is also collaborating with AIDS vaccine programs internationally to coordinate the effort.

Safety Issues

Because HIV targets the immune system itself, vaccines that contain HIV components may pose unusual risks. For example, HIV has a number of immunogenic regions—epitopes—that are homologous to epitopes on human immune cells. Accordingly, there is at least a theoretical potential for vaccine-induced antibodies that react with host immune cells and inhibit immune function or induce autoreactive mechanisms.

Another potential risk is enhancement of infection. With ADCC, the Fab portion of an antibody produced in response to a vaccine will attach to viral antigen presented on the surface of an infected host cell. The Fc portion may bind to an Fc receptor on a killer cell, which will then lyse the infected cell. Macrophages also have a number of Fc receptors, however, and HIV infects those cells. Binding of HIV to a macrophage via antibody may not result in destruction of the virus but rather facilitate its entry into the macrophage.

Enhancement occurs in a variety of viral diseases. Kittens immunized with inactivated feline leukemia virus and then challenged with live virus have shown enhanced disease compared with unimmunized controls. Dengue fever can occur with particular severity in human infants with maternal antibody titers that have declined to low levels.

Enhancement has been demonstrated in vitro with HIV. If the virus is placed into macrophage cultures containing low titers of antibody against HIV, the result is increased infection of macrophages. Researchers are currently exploring the question of whether enhancement can occur in vivo. Macaques immunized and then infected have not demonstrated evidence of in vivo enhancement, even if low levels of antibody are produced.

Approaches to AIDS Vaccines

Various approaches are being explored for the development of AIDS vaccines. One that is not currently being actively developed, although it is used for a variety of other diseases, is the use of live attenuated virus. Such vaccines can induce both humoral and cellular immunity, and vaccines containing whole virus have the advantage of presenting antigens to the host in a form equivalent to that of natural infection. Live attenuated virus vaccines can produce severe reactions in immunodeficient recipients, however—a particular concern with HIV, in view of the frequency of immunodeficiency in developing nations where AIDS is epidemic. The risk of incorporation into host cell DNA is also great.

Vaccines containing whole killed virus have also been successful against other diseases and are being evaluated for AIDS. Those containing killed HIV are now undergoing clinical trials in HIV-infected individuals, in efforts to slow the progression to AIDS. With killed vaccines, of course, the goal is to destroy the functional capacity of viral nucleic acid, while maintaining the conformational integrity of viral proteins and thus their ability to stimulate specific immune responses. A paramount concern with these vaccines will be safety.

A newer approach to vaccine development, which capitalizes on modern molecular biology, is the use of live recombinant viruses. Genes encoding for HIV antigens can be spliced into the genetic structure of an unrelated virus, such as vaccinia, which is then used as a vector. Replication of the carrier virus results in the production of large amounts of HIV antigens—thus potentially producing greater immunogenicity than do nonreplicating vaccines. Since recombinant viruses do not contain the genes for HIV replication, there is no risk of integration and persistence of HIV genetic material in host cell DNA. Recombinant techniques have also been used to produce vaccines containing pseudovirions, which include viral nucleic acids but have mutations in the viral proteins that bind RNA and so are nonfunctional.

The first human immunizations with a candidate AIDS vaccine, performed in 1986 in healthy HIV-seronegative volunteers in Zaire and France, used a recombinant vaccinia virus expressing the HIV envelope glycoprotein gp160 (Figure 2). The vaccine was well tolerated and induced both antibody and cell-mediated immune responses, but at low

Figure 2. Potential Immunogens Produced by the HIV Genome

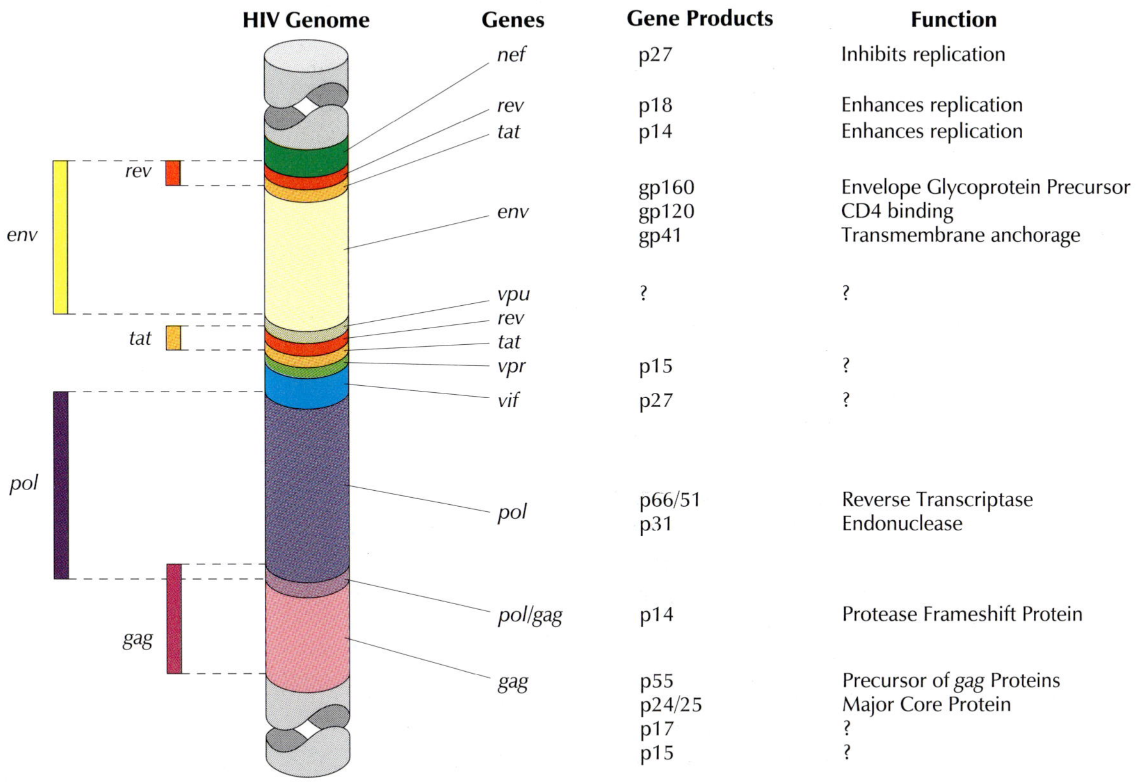
HIV Genome
Genes
Gene Products
Function
nef
p27
Inhibits replication
rev
p18
Enhances replication
tat
p14
Enhances replication
env
gp160
Envelope Glycoprotein Precursor
gp120
CD4 binding
gp41
Transmembrane anchorage
vpu
?
?
rev
tat
vpr
p15
?
vif
p27
?
pol
p66/51
Reverse Transcriptase
p31
Endonuclease
pol/gag
p14
Protease Frameshift Protein
gag
p55
Precursor of gag Proteins
p24/25
Major Core Protein
p17
?
p15
?
env
rev
tat
pol
gag

levels. In an expansion of the study, those responses were successfully boosted by addition of killed autologous cells previously infected with the recombinant virus, followed by purified recombinant gp160. Although such a strategy is logistically too complex to be used on a large scale, the studies suggest that similar booster strategies may be effective.

Such strategies may be necessary because the humoral immune responses generated by candidate vaccines are generally weaker than those produced by other viral immunogens. Potentiation of immune responses through the use of adjuvants is also being investigated.

Two clinical trials of recombinant vaccinia virus containing the gene for the HIV envelope have been conducted in the United States. Vaccine recipients who were not previously immune to vaccinia mounted strong T-cell proliferative responses. Researchers are now studying recombinant vaccines using a number of other vectors, including adenoviruses, poliovirus, BCG, and herpesviruses.

On another front, the NIAID and the AIDS Vaccine Clinical Trials Network recently reported phase 1 results with a recombinant gp160-subunit candidate vaccine in healthy, HIV-negative subjects. The preparation, which was administered in two doses on four occasions, was well tolerated and frequently immunogenic after the third and fourth administrations (Figure 3).

A number of vaccines containing synthetic peptide antigens are under investigation. The peptides can be selected to include epitopes for stimulating humoral and cellular immunity, to exclude immunosuppressive epitopes, and to be free of viral nucleic acid. The relative immunogenicity of peptides compared with whole viral proteins is unclear. One such synthetic peptide, designated HGP-30, is derived from the HIV p17 core protein. It is now being studied in a clinical trial of HIV-infected men in the United Kingdom.

The use of genetically engineered purified HIV antigens is a potentially promising approach to AIDS vaccines. It has a successful precedent in recombinant hepatitis B vaccine. One question about recombinant vaccines is whether the system used to express HIV antigen affects the antigen's immunogenic potential. Several expression systems are being used for production of HIV antigens, including insect cells, *E. coli*, yeast, and mammalian cells. Those systems differ in their ability to duplicate the carbohydrate portion of HIV glycoproteins, with mammalian cells providing the best match. Comparison of the efficacy of vaccines using the same antigen expressed by different systems should determine whether such glycosylation is an important factor.

A second question is which antigen or antigens should be chosen. In selecting HIV gene products for subunit vaccines, the major focus has been on products of the *env* gene—gp160, gp120, and gp41. Those are glycoproteins of HIV's lipid envelope (gp160 is the precursor of gp120 and gp41). They are therefore exposed to host immune defense mechanisms and contain both neutralizing and T-cell epitopes. Gene products of proteins located within the whole virion are also being used in can-

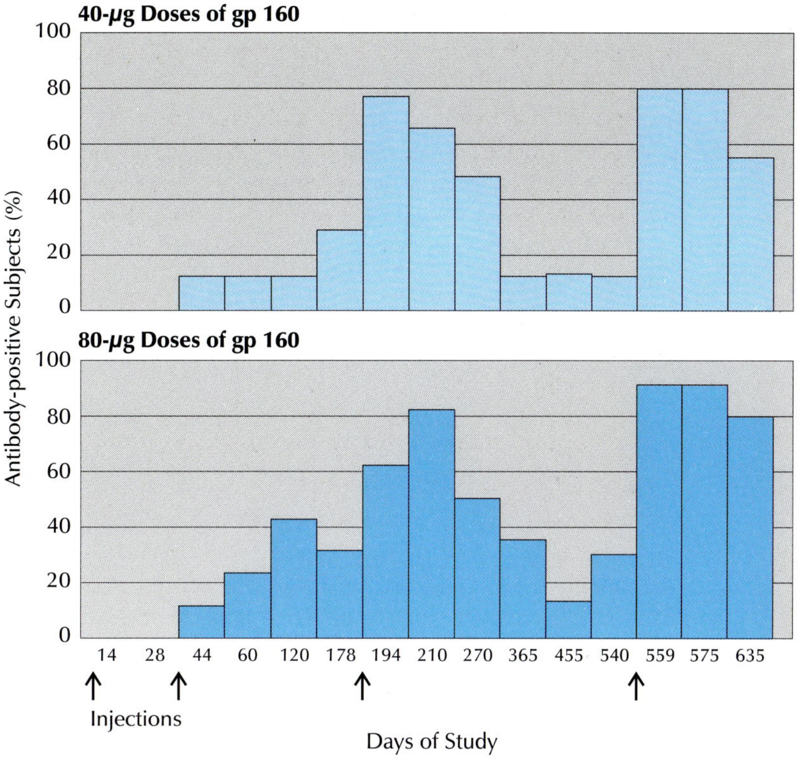

Figure 3 In a phase 1 trial, Raphael Dolin and co-workers of the AIDS Vaccine Clinical Trials Network reported no serious toxicities and frequent antibody responses with 40-μg (top) or 80-μg doses (bottom) of a recombinant gp160 vaccine in healthy seronegative subjects (administrations indicated by arrows). With both dosages, responses were commonly weak on Western blot assays and were first noted after the second dose. The frequency of response markedly increased after the third dose, subsequently declined, and then rose after the fourth dose. (Adapted from Ann Intern Med 114:119, 1991)

didate vaccines, however, because they may be expressed on the surface of infected cells and therefore may be integral to induction of host immune responses. Experiments to date have not proved that any one HIV gene product is critical for protection. It may be that an effective subunit vaccine requires combinations of viral proteins to stimulate effective immunity.

One region that may be important for inducing neutralizing antibodies is the V3 loop of gp120, the glycoprotein that binds to the CD4 receptor, which is the primary attachment site of HIV on CD4 lymphocytes (Figure 4). The V3 loop, however, has turned out to be one of the most variable of all the regions of the virus; study of numerous HIV isolates has shown wide differences in the amino acid sequences of the loop. That, of course, is not coincidental; the variability is a survival advantage for the virus. The good news is that the crown of the loop is not as variable as the other portions and appears to be among the most important for inducing neutralizing immune responses. Consequently, it is possible that the problem of

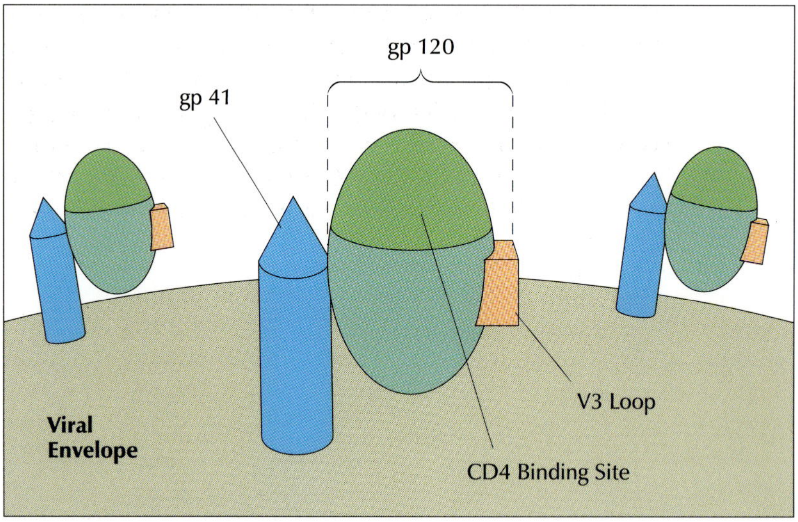

Figure 4 HIV's envelope glycoprotein gp120, which is associated with the transmembrane glycoprotein gp41, contains two epitopes that have attracted interest as targets for vaccines. One is the CD4 binding site, thought to mediate attachment of HIV-infected cells to several uninfected cell populations. The other is a region of gp120 known as the V3 loop, which may be involved in events subsequent to attachment. Although highly variable among HIV isolates, the V3 loop appears to be strongly immunogenic.

variability may be overcome through use of a cocktail containing highly prevalent isolates, much as multivalent vaccines are now used against viral diseases such as polio.

An early clue that antibodies directed against the gp120 region of the viral envelope may correlate with immunity emerged from studies of HIV transmission from mothers to newborns. These studies have also suggested a novel use for AIDS vaccines. Overall, approximately one third of babies born to infected mothers are themselves infected. Three independent analyses have shown that infants whose mothers have antibodies to gp120 are at significantly lower risk of infection than infants whose mothers lack those antibodies. More precise techniques used in two analyses pinpointed portions of the V3 loop as the critical site. If confirmed, such observations raise the possibility that vaccination of infected women with V3-loop determinants, or perhaps those of the entire envelope, may induce immune responses that prevent vertical transmission of HIV.

Vaccines as Therapy

Another possible use for AIDS vaccines is as therapy in persons already infected with HIV. The usual long delay between initial infection and development of AIDS suggests that host immune defenses may control the infection for a time but are eventually overwhelmed. Jonas Salk has hypothesized that boosting protective immune responses against

HIV during the asymptomatic period might reduce the viral burden and thereby prevent progression to AIDS. Salk and colleagues have begun testing that hypothesis, using HIV that has been killed with gamma radiation and depleted of gp120. Taking different routes in the same direction, other investigators, including Robert Redfield and his group at Walter Reed Army Medical Center, Washington, D.C., are studying recombinant gp160 or other recombinant envelope vaccines against established HIV infection.

The use of AIDS vaccines as therapy, of course, confronts with particular force the issue of whether it is possible to mobilize the immune system against a pathogen that infects the immune system itself. Even before their CD4 lymphocyte counts begin to fall, HIV-infected persons may have sustained imperceptible but significant immune damage. For example, the virus may have modified antigen presentation by macrophages such that vaccine response is no longer optimal and therefore not protective. Nonetheless, preliminary safety and immunogenicity studies of the Salk HIV vaccine in patients with asymptomatic and early symptomatic HIV infection have been encouraging. Recently, the Food and Drug Administration approved expanded clinical trials of the vaccine.

Anti-idiotype antibodies constitute another approach to AIDS vaccines (Figure 5). Such antibodies recognize idiotypic determinants that identify the variable regions of other antibodies. Anti-idiotype antibodies specific for the CD4 molecule may thus serve as CD4 surrogates. Studies in mice have shown that anti-idiotype antibodies generated in response to an anti-CD4 antibody are capable of binding and neutralizing genetically divergent isolates of HIV.

Potential drawbacks to the approach include the possibility that there are multiple HIV recognition sites on CD4, and that inoculation with anti-CD4 antibodies may induce immunosuppression, given the central role that the CD4 lymphocyte plays in the orchestration of T-lymphocyte helper/inducer immune responses. Those issues are currently being addressed in preclinical studies.

V3-loop anti-idiotypic antibodies are also under study as a vaccine. If effective, they would induce antibodies that bind the loop, yet avoid the risk of exposing vaccine recipients to viral material.

It is likely that more than one vaccine will ultimately be considered for large-scale trials, because of the different applications envisioned for AIDS vaccines. For example, recombinant vectors that are suitable for priming cellular immune responses in uninfected subjects may cause disease in HIV-seropositive subjects. On the other hand, peptides that boost immune responses in seropositive subjects may not elicit a primary response in seronegative ones.

Difficulties of Vaccine Trials

The testing of AIDS vaccines in humans poses several scientific issues and problems. What, for instance, should be the end point of clinical vac-

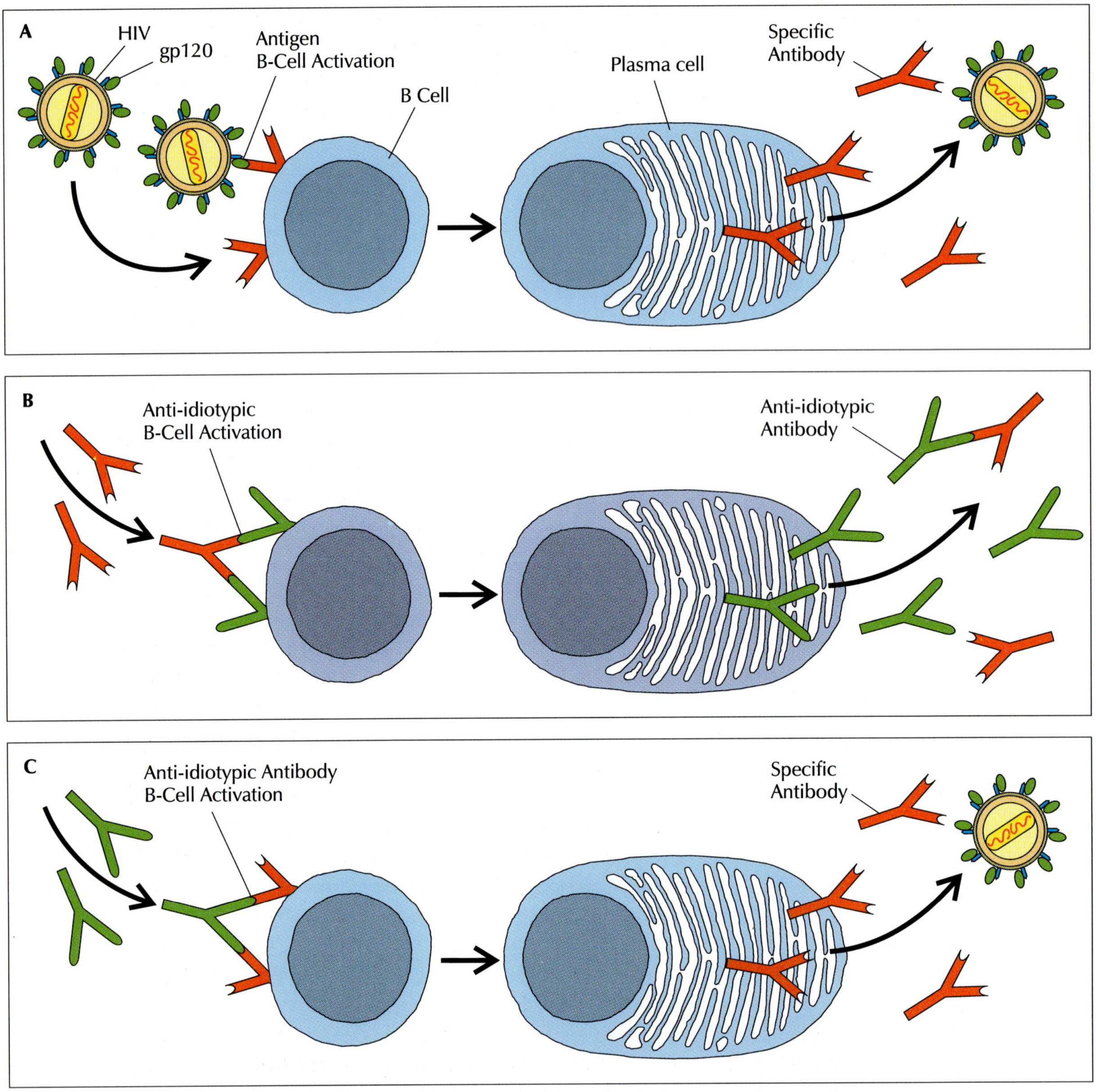

Figure 5 Anti-idiotype antibodies afford an approach to AIDS vaccine development. They would serve as immunizing surrogates for HIV antigenic determinants, such as gp120 (or gp120's V3 loop). An antibody directed against such antigen (A) would stimulate production of a second antibody directed against an idiotypic determinant on the original antibody molecule (B). If the anti-idiotype antibody is then used as an immunogen, it would activate the same B-cell clones as the antigen itself, stimulating an immune response against the virus (C).

cine trials—protection against initiation of infection, establishment of infection, or clinical illness?

There is no evidence that any vaccine can prevent initial infection with a virus. In a person who has been vaccinated against poliomyelitis, measles, or influenza, subsequent exposure to specific virus results in a subclinical infection that the immune system recognizes and quickly eliminates. It has been argued, however, that the ability to prevent initial infection might be a prerequisite for an effective AIDS vaccine. Unlike poliovirus, measles virus, or influenza virus, HIV can persist in latent form in the host cell DNA, so an immunologic response might not clear the virus from the blood.

The latent viral genetic material can now be detected with a new laboratory technique, polymerase chain reaction (PCR). Epidemiologic studies involving PCR have produced mixed results to date. Some subjects with positive PCR studies have subsequently progressed to clinical illness; others have not. The frequency with which seronegative persons may go on to have disease after HIV is detected by PCR is unknown. Our knowledge has not yet caught up with our technology in this respect. Most likely, preventing establishment of infection will be considered an end point for the first few vaccine efficacy trials. However, if we presume that a positive reaction on PCR testing indicates infection, which can theoretically be transmitted to another person in that latent form, a vaccine that prevented the establishment of infection but permitted the provirus to enter host cells might not, from a public health perspective, significantly inhibit virus transmission.

If preventing initial infection is impossible, an alternative end point for vaccine trials is maintaining the virus in latent form. At present we have no way of knowing whether that is an acceptable outcome. Even if it were acceptable, it is not very practical, given the length of HIV's latency period; such a trial might require 10 years or more to complete.

As with many other sexually transmitted diseases, AIDS vaccine trials involve complex informed-consent issues: the obligation to counsel subjects about avoiding high-risk behavior for HIV infection, and the mission to evaluate the efficacy of the vaccine. If counseling uniformly eliminated high-risk behavior, a vaccine trial would be impossible. In real life, designers of such studies can model them using historical estimates of the percentage of subjects in whom counseling will fail (despite all attempts) and then plan the trial size accordingly.

Recruitment of volunteers for vaccine trials promises to be difficult. Subjects will have to be assured that complete confidentiality will be maintained because they may be identified as persons at risk for HIV infection.

Also, trial subjects who mount effective immune responses to some candidate vaccines will then have positive results on ELISA tests for HIV antibody; subjects receiving vaccines with multiple antigens might also have a positive Western blot. They might therefore be subject to the social stigma and discrimination associated with HIV infection. Although such subjects could be given identification cards to document their participation in a vaccine trial, they might still encounter difficulties in donating blood, obtaining insurance, traveling internationally, or entering the military or foreign service.

A strategy now under consideration is the inclusion of a marker vaccine against an unrelated substance. Antibodies against that substance would be evidence that HIV seropositivity was vaccine induced. Even that, however, does not address the risk that a subject in whom vaccination is ineffective might subsequently become infected and capable of transmitting the disease. Distinguishing protective from infective seropositivity is less of a concern for vaccine researchers. They can use molecular tests to ascertain whether the antibodies match the isolate used in the vaccine, or they can check for live virus.

Spin-offs

The effort to develop AIDS vaccines could conceivably do as much for the development of vaccines against other viruses as for the battle against AIDS. Approaches such as synthetic peptides, vectors, and anti-idiotypes may find ready application against other viruses. For example, vectors promise to be useful for the production of combination vaccines that can provide simultaneous protection against several viral pathogens.

Thus, research efforts in AIDS vaccine development need to be intensified not only because of the immediate public health priority of preventing and controlling HIV infection but also because of the potential for preventing and controlling other infectious diseases.

SELECTED READING

Koff WC, Hoth DF: Development and testing of AIDS vaccines. Science 241:426, 1988

Koff WC, Fauci AS: Human trials of AIDS vaccines: Current status and future directions. AIDS 1989 3(suppl 1):S125, 1989

Scott CF Jr et al: Human monoclonal antibody that recognizes the V3 region of human immunodeficiency virus gp120 and neutralizes the human T-lymphotropic virus type IIIMN strain. Proc Natl Acad Sci USA 87:8597, 1990

Verdin E et al: Identification and characterization of an enhancer in the coding region of the genome of human immunodeficiency virus type 1. Proc Natl Acad Sci USA 87:4874, 1990

Barrett N et al: Large-scale production and purification of a vaccinia recombinant-derived HIV-1 gp160 and analysis of its immunogenicity. AIDS Res Hum Retroviruses 5:159, 1989

Vaccine Adjuvant Research May Hold Key to Successful AIDS Vaccine Development. AIDS Research Exchange, September/October 1989, pp 1–8 (Technical Resources, Inc, Rockville, Md)

7 HIV Infection in Maternal and Pediatric Patients

CATHERINE M. WILFERT *Duke University*

Although children constitute only 2% of the recognized cases of AIDS in the United States, the incidence of HIV infection in children is rising rapidly. Within the next few years an additional 10,000 to 20,000 cases are expected. That projection reflects the spread of HIV among women of childbearing age (Figure 1), who contract the infection from infected sex partners or intravenous drug use with contaminated needles and then transmit infection vertically. From 1988 to 1989, AIDS in women and vertically acquired AIDS in children rose 36% and 38%, respectively, increasing more steeply than any other category of AIDS cases. Less than 1% of AIDS cases are found at the far end of the pediatric spectrum—the adolescent years—but the rapid increase in AIDS among young adults indicates that HIV infection is acquired more often during adolescence than the reported number of AIDS cases would suggest.

AIDS in children differs from AIDS in adults in several important respects. Vertical transmission of HIV infection and the immaturity of the infant's immune system alter the natural history of the disease and affect medical management. The provision of medical care and social support to these children is often complicated by socioeconomic disadvantages and by the fact that the mothers (and sometimes other household members) are themselves ill with the disease.

In the United States today, HIV-infected women of childbearing age predominantly are poor, are black or Hispanic, and live in the inner city, particularly in the Northeast and Florida. Seropositivity is increasing in rural areas of the southeastern states, however. In our clinics in North Carolina, approximately half of patients appear to have acquired their infection locally, which suggests that the behavior facilitating the spread of the disease extended from adjacent metropolitan areas some years ago. Since such behavior presumably is not restricted to the Southeast, it is reasonable to assume that the pattern will eventually be repeated in other rural areas of the United States.

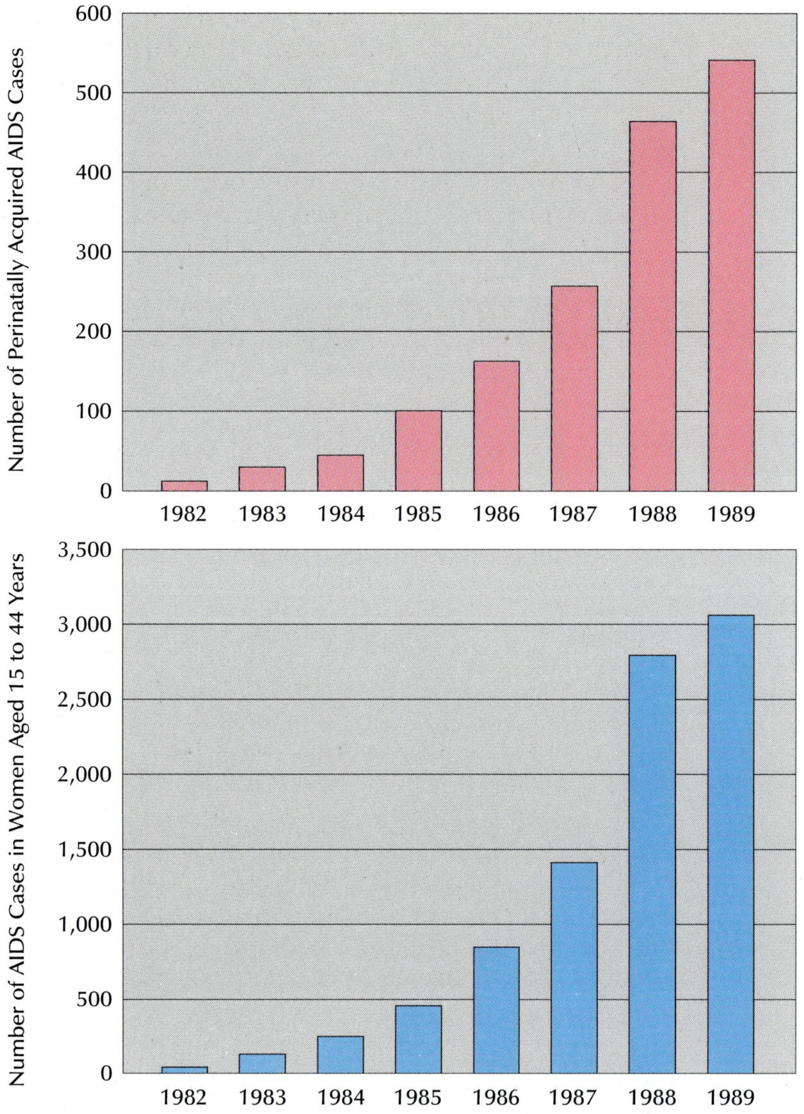

Figure 1 The annual number of perinatally acquired AIDS cases reported in the United States rose steadily during the 1980s, from a handful to several hundred (top). That trend paralleled an increase in the annual number of AIDS cases that occurred in women of reproductive age (15 to 44).

In North Carolina, and conceivably elsewhere as well, about two thirds of the HIV-seropositive mothers in whom the source of infection can be identified apparently acquired their infection through IV drug use. In about one third, the infection can be traced to heterosexual transmission, usually from IV drug-using partners.

No significant influence of pregnancy on the course of HIV infection in the mother has been demonstrated. On the other hand, infants born to seropositive mothers in developing nations are likely to be small for gestational age and have high mortality in the first two years of life.

HIV appears to be transmitted relatively inefficiently from mother to offspring. Reported vertical transmission rates have ranged as high as 65%, but prospective studies from Europe and the United States suggest rates of 30% or lower. For instance, the European Collaborative Study recently reported a 13% rate of vertical HIV transmission. This study involved women known to be seropositive at or before delivery. Uniform screening of all pregnant women was not used. Although the study was well designed, the possibility must be considered that its relatively low transmission rate reflects selection of a population of HIV-infected women who transmit infection at a lower rate than the entire population.

Transmission rates, for example, may correlate with the stage of maternal illness. In studies from Africa and France, women with advanced disease were most likely to transmit infection to their babies. Those studies were dependent on selective CD4 assessment and cord blood cultures of a small subpopulation. It is logical, however, that more-advanced disease and greater viral burden would enhance transmission. As increasing numbers of women with advanced disease come under study in the United States and Europe, more reliable data should become available.

Even if confirmed, however, such a correlation would have no predictive significance in individual cases. Furthermore, a woman may transmit HIV to her infant despite being asymptomatic and having a CD4 count greater than 400. Higher transmission rates have been reported among women who lacked antibody responses to HIV glycoprotein 120 epitopes, which may be important in HIV binding to CD4-bearing cells. Unfortunately, the correlation did not rest simply on the absence of gp120 antibodies but on that of high-affinity antibodies, and other laboratories using the same sera have not been able to confirm those results.

Mechanism(s) and Manifestations

The mechanism of HIV transmission to the fetus or newborn is unknown. Transmission has occurred in utero, and it is strongly suspected that this may occur around the time of delivery. Vaginal secretions, for example, have been found to contain HIV. The virus has been cultured from fetuses aborted between nine and 20 weeks' gestation. It has been isolated from or demonstrated by the polymerase chain reaction technique in neonatal cord blood lymphocytes and newborn peripheral blood mononuclear cells in up to 50% of infants ultimately shown to be infected. It is hoped that the failure to detect infection uniformly means these infants are not infected in utero but have acquired virus around the time of delivery. This might provide an opportunity to interrupt transmission.

Clinical manifestations of AIDS in children are listed in Table 1. Some investigators have posited the existence of a dysmorphic syndrome in HIV-infected neonates, characterized by growth retardation, microcephaly, and abnormal facies. Such a syndrome would be evidence of in utero HIV transmission. The norms used to establish facial abnor-

Table 1. Clinical Manifestations of AIDS in Children

Features More Common in Children than in Adults

- Recurrent bacterial infections
- Chronic interstitial pneumonitis
- Failure to thrive
- Parotitis

Features Common in Children and Adults

- Non-CNS opportunistic infections (e.g., PCP)
- Chronic mucocutaneous candidiasis
- Neurologic abnormalities
- Chronic or recurrent diarrhea
- Chronic or recurrent fevers
- Diffuse adenopathy
- Hepatosplenomegaly
- Chronic eczemoid rash
- Progressive renal disease
- Cardiomyopathy

Features More Common in Adults than in Children

- Neoplasms (including Kaposi sarcoma and lymphomas)
- Opportunistic infections of the central nervous system

malities were those for white rather than black or Hispanic infants, however. Furthermore, a study of African mothers who were not drug users found no dysmorphic features in infected infants. The dysmorphic syndrome, if it exists at all, may be related to drug use rather than to HIV infection.

The risk of contracting HIV infection from breast-feeding is unknown. Breast-feeding was the likely route of transmission reported in infants who acquired infection during or after delivery. However, studies from developing countries do not show increased transmission rates in breast-feeding seropositive women compared with non-breast-feeding seropositive women. Because HIV can be isolated from lymphocytes in breast milk from seropositive mothers, such women in the United States and other developed countries are generally advised not to breast-feed their infants. In developing countries, breast-feeding is essential for optimal nutrition and survival and continues to be recommended regardless of HIV infection in the mother.

A possible clue to the timing of vertical transmission can be found in the natural history of pediatric AIDS. About 20% of infected infants become symptomatic during the first few months of life. Those infants tend to follow an acute course and do badly. It seems reasonable to speculate that their disease rapidly progresses because the virus was transmitted through the placenta, perhaps early in the first trimester. Presumably, infection was acquired before the thymus was fully developed, and virus may have been incubating for as much as six months before birth.

The majority of vertically infected infants progress to AIDS more gradually. Mathematical modeling suggests that AIDS develops in infected infants at a rate of approximately 10% each year, with a median age at diagnosis of three years or older; by age 10 almost all have AIDS. The slower course may reflect infection acquired around the time of delivery. Efforts to detect HIV within the first few weeks of life are unsuccessful in 50% of infected infants, which would be consistent with recently acquired infection and a light viral burden.

In the United States, vertical transmission now accounts for more than 80% of AIDS cases in children under the age of 13. Infection in the remaining 20% was largely transmitted through transfusions of blood and blood products. Screening and other safety measures instituted since 1985 have virtually eliminated those sources of HIV infection, but new cases continue to be identified because the mean incubation period in transfusion-acquired or coagulation factor–acquired AIDS is estimated to range from 3½ to 10 years. Maternal-to-infant transmission is now responsible for almost all pediatric HIV infection.

The AIDS Clinical Trials Group is initiating a large study (ACTG protocol 076) to investigate the possibility of interrupting vertical transmission with zidovudine. Seropositive women with CD4 counts greater than 200 will be randomized for treatment during pregnancy, and the drug will be continued in infants for the first six weeks of life. Zidovudine will not be started in the first trimester and cannot be expected to stop all transmission. Should zidovudine reduce transmission rates, the trial may establish that significant transmission occurs around the time of delivery.

Women who enter the health care system only when in active labor have not had the advantage of prenatal care for themselves or access to specific antiretroviral therapy or supportive care for HIV infection. This adds further urgency to the need for prenatal care in the poor. Women will avail themselves of such care, provided it is accessible, of good quality, and affordable. At Lincoln Community Health Care Center (a federally funded facility in downtown Durham serving an indigent population), 90% of pregnant women are seen before the third trimester. Preventive medicine tends to be eminently cost-effective, and the potential is particularly great with a disease as expensive as AIDS. The annual cost of treating a vertically infected infant on Medicaid has been estimated at $18,000 to $42,000.

Diagnosis

Vertically transmitted HIV infection presents unique diagnostic difficulties. Although most infants born to HIV-seropositive women are not infected with HIV, all are seropositive at birth and in the first months of life because maternal antibodies to HIV are transmitted across the placenta. Loss of antibody and consistent seronegativity at 15 months of age indicate that the infant is not infected.

ELISA and Western blot assays are routinely used in these infants to confirm that HIV antibody is present. The Western blot could have a further diagnostic use: If analysis showed that specific antibody against a given viral protein is present in the infant's serum but not in maternal serum, one could be fairly confident that the infant was infected and was making the antibody. That does not happen very often, however, and this approach is impractical for large-scale use.

Among various laboratory tests available (Table 2), the most reliable

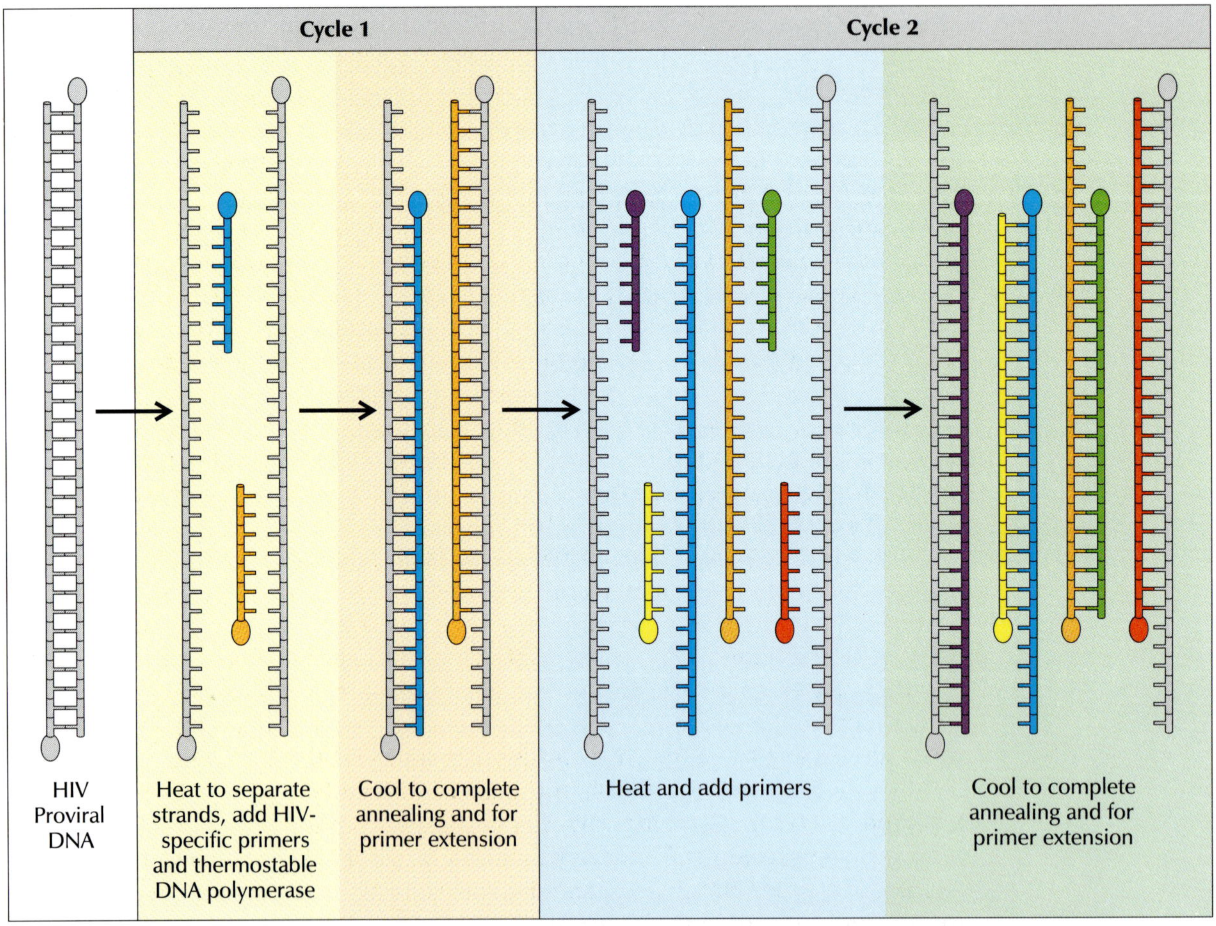

Figure 2 The polymerase chain reaction technique offers a highly accurate means for early diagnosis of HIV infection. DNA from peripheral blood leukocytes is cyclically heated and cooled in the presence of thermostable DNA polymerase and complementary nucleotide sequences (primers) specific for HIV. When HIV proviral DNA is present, heating induces strand separation, and cooling allows the primers to anneal to the separated strands; DNA polymerase then catalyzes addition to the primers of nucleotides complementary to the strands (primer extension). By this process, the number of DNA strands containing the proviral sequence doubles at the end of each cycle. The cycling is repeated many times until HIV proviral DNA has been amplified at least 10^5-fold.

Table 2. Laboratory Studies for Diagnosis of HIV Infection in Newborns, Infants, and Children

HIV cultures (with peripheral blood mononuclear cells and, if available, plasma)

Polymerase chain reaction testing with peripheral blood leukocytes

HIV antibody on ELISA or Western blot*

Serum or plasma p24 antigen

CBC and total lymphocyte count†

CD3, CD4, and CD8 counts and percentages; CD4/CD8 ratio†

Quantitative serum IgG, IgM, and IgA determinations†

*Positive results in newborns denote maternal infection

†Nondiagnostic in newborns but provides baseline immunologic data

for early diagnosis are viral culture and polymerase chain reaction (PCR) testing. Unfortunately, HIV culture may take as long as four weeks, and both tests require laboratory expertise not yet widely available.

PCR detects proviral DNA sequences of HIV. The viral DNA is amplified as much as a millionfold (Figure 2). The exquisite sensitivity means that any contaminating DNA that is amplified will also be detected. Consequently, strict quality control is essential for achieving reliable results with PCR. Research firms have developed methods of reducing the number of false-positives, which is essential if PCR is to become a routine procedure. In the meantime, the results of properly performed PCR assays correlate well with HIV cultures. With both methods, approximately half of infected infants will be identified in the newborn period, and most will be detected by three to six months of age.

In the future, IgA antibody may be the key to early diagnosis. Unlike IgG, IgA does not cross the placenta. Specific IgA-HIV antibody is produced by the infant and not transplacentally acquired. Thus, IgA-HIV seropositivity defines an infected infant. In several experimental series, most infected infants have demonstrated HIV-specific IgA antibody in the first six months of life. An IgA antibody assay is not yet commercially available as testing in sufficient numbers of infants is still in progress.

Although most HIV-infected infants are clinically and immunologically normal at birth, within months they may manifest immunologic abnormalities suggesting infection. As in adults, levels of CD4 lymphocytes decline as infection progresses, and comparisons must be made to age-appropriate normal values (Table 3).

The levels are usually quite high at birth and decline gradually to adult values. CD4 counts in healthy infants may be as high as 3,000 or more. Counts of less than 1,500 in the first year, less than 750 between one and two years, less than 500 between two and six years, and less than 200 after six years have been established as values indicating risk of *Pneumocystis carinii* pneumonia (PCP) in HIV-infected children. These values signify that severe immunologic compromise exists.

Table 3. Age-Adjusted CD4 Values in Healthy Children and Adults (Data from CDC)

	Children (Age in Months)				*Adults*
	1–6	*7–12*	*13–24*	*25–74*	
Numbers Tested	106	28	46	29	327
Absolute CD4 Count					
Median (cells/mm^3)	3,211	3,128	2,601	1,668	1,027
5th–95th percentile	1,153–5,285	967–5,289	739–4,463	505–2,831	237–1,817
CD4 Percentage					
Median	51.6	47.9	45.8	42.1	50.9
5th–95th percentile	36.3–67.1	32.8–63.0	31.2–60.4	32.2–52.0	34.7–67.1
CD4/CD8 Ratio					
Median	2.2	2.1	2.0	1.4	1.7
5th–95th percentile	0.9–3.5	0.8–3.4	0.6–3.4	0.7–2.1	0.4–3.0

Another indirect marker of HIV infection is elevation of serum immune globulins. Polyclonal hypergammaglobulinemia occurs in about 80% of infected children, often in the first months of life. Less commonly (in about 10% of cases), infected infants will have hypogammaglobulinemia.

Clinical Course

As noted, vertically transmitted AIDS tends to follow either of two courses. In early-onset disease, severe immunodeficiency usually develops rapidly in the first year of life. This population presents with PCP, and mortality is high; median survival is one to four months after onset of the pneumonia.

Although the clinical course in infants often includes wasting syndrome and encephalopathy, PCP is the dominant illness. It is more often fatal in infants than in adults and is the major cause of death in the first year of life in HIV-infected infants. PCP is more severe in these infants perhaps in part because it is a primary infection. Normal, HIV-negative persons have serologic evidence of primary infection with *P. carinii* in early childhood years and do not have clinically significant illness. There is a paucity of information elucidating the elements of the immune response that enable immunocompetent hosts to control the infection. However, immunocompromised patients with isolated anti-

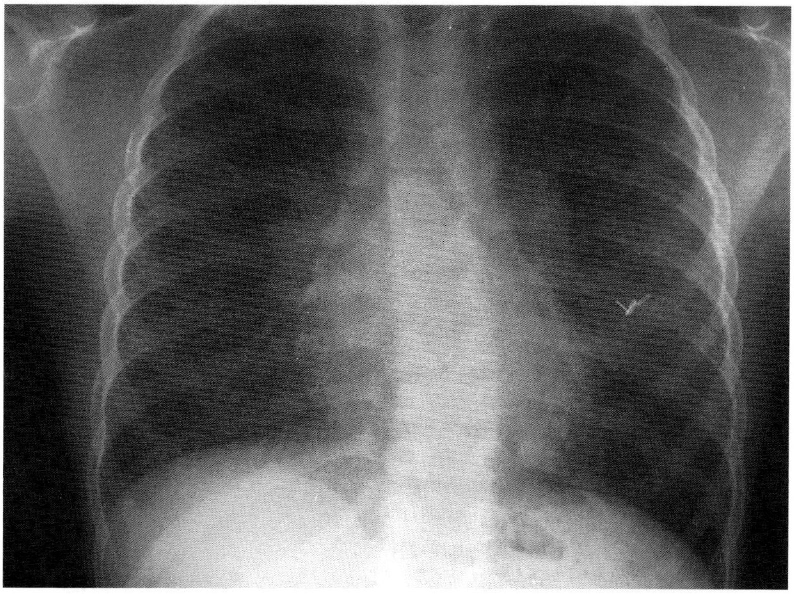

Figure 3 A common presenting disease in children with vertically acquired HIV infection is lymphoid interstitial pneumonitis (LIP), in which a chest x-ray typically shows a reticulonodular pattern, sometimes with hilar adenopathy. LIP often manifests at about age two in the clinical context of tachypnea, cough, wheezing, and hypoxemia. Definitive diagnosis requires lung biopsy.

body deficits do not have the same risk of PCP as do patients with T-lymphocyte deficits, suggesting that host cell–mediated immunity is of great importance.

In children with late-onset HIV infection, many remain asymptomatic for years, and others gradually manifest signs and symptoms of infection. The clinical picture in this group often includes evidence of lymphoproliferative processes, such as hepatosplenomegaly, lymphadenopathy, or parotid gland enlargement.

A common lymphoproliferative process in this group, and one that is virtually never seen in adults with AIDS, is pulmonary lymphoid hyperplasia, or lymphoid interstitial pneumonitis (LIP). Unlike Pneumocystis pneumonia, which is usually diagnosed in the first year of life, LIP is typically identified in children who are about two years old. Affected children initially have asymptomatic chronic pulmonary infiltration, then slowly manifest clinical symptoms that include tachypnea, cough, wheezing, and hypoxemia. Digital clubbing is common in advanced cases. The chest x-ray typically shows a reticulonodular pattern, sometimes with hilar adenopathy (Figure 3). Lung biopsy is necessary for definitive diagnosis, however. A diagnostic approach to LIP is shown in Figure 4.

Children who present with LIP have a predictably longer life expectancy than those who present with PCP or encephalopathy. Mortality

Figure 4. An Approach to the Child with Evidence of LIP on X-ray

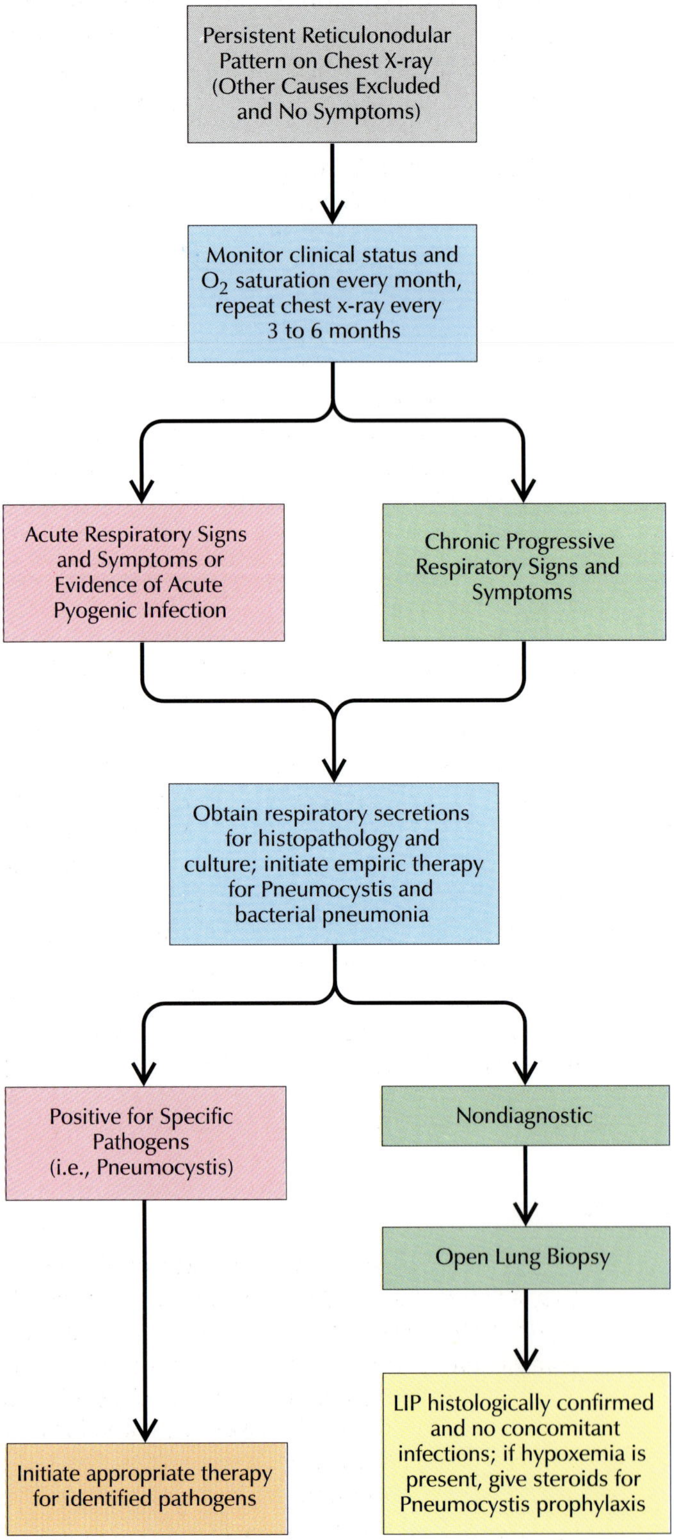

one year after diagnosis is approximately 30%, compared with about 75% for children presenting with PCP. It is tempting to link the greater survival with the high incidence of Epstein-Barr virus infection in children with LIP. EBV is known to stimulate lymphoproliferation. The question has been raised whether interaction between the two viruses is favorable to the host for a time.

Concurrent EBV infection could help explain why LIP sometimes progresses to neoplastic disease—polyclonal B-cell lymphoproliferative disorder. Epstein-Barr virus infection is clearly associated with B-cell malignancies in bone marrow transplant patients who are heavily immunosuppressed. A polyclonal B-cell lymphoproliferative disorder has not been common in children with LIP, however, and the majority of these children die of opportunistic infections.

Recurrent bacterial infections, ranging from persistent otitis media to overwhelming bacterial meningitis, are very common in HIV-infected children. Approximately 80% of those who fit the CDC classification for symptomatic HIV infection have elevated immunoglobulin levels—in itself an indication of impaired immune regulation—and many have reduced ability to make specific antibody in response to primary exposure to antigens. Until the age of 18 months to two years, even normal children may be immunologically incapable of recognizing many capsular polysaccharides as antigens to which they should mount a response—which is why, for example, *Hemophilus influenzae* type B is a common invasive pathogen in that age group. Among HIV-infected children, that deficiency is enhanced and persists longer.

HIV central nervous system disease is more common in children than in adults. In most series, 50% to 90% of infected children have clinical evidence of HIV-related CNS disease. Among infants and toddlers, failure to achieve or loss of normal developmental milestones constitutes the most common clinical manifestation of infection. Children who had apparently been developing normally may begin to lose verbal and motor skills. Neurodevelopmental deterioration is often accompanied by overt neurologic abnormalities and sometimes by changes in EEG and head CT scans or MRI. Cerebrospinal fluid abnormalities do not accurately predict CNS compromise. Opportunistic infections of the central nervous system are rare in children compared with adults.

Treatment

Investigational agents are traditionally tested first in adults, before they are incorporated into pediatric practice. That was true as therapy against HIV was initiated. The number of HIV-infected adults is far greater than that of infected infants and children. The efficacy of zidovudine was first shown in a randomized placebo-controlled trial in symptomatic adults. Zidovudine was approved for therapy of HIV infection in adults in 1987. It was not until 1990 that the drug was approved for use in children with the same disease. We are now able to obtain initial toxicity data for promising antiretroviral agents in adults and proceed immediately to preliminary studies in children. Effective therapy that is appropriately studied and found to be adequately tolerated and safe should become available for HIV-infected adults and children at the same time.

In August 1989, studies demonstrated that treatment with zidovudine could significantly slow the progression to AIDS in asymptomatic or minimally symptomatic adults, if the drug was given when the CD4 count fell below 500. Presumably, that approach would also be effective in children, albeit at an age-adjusted CD4 count.

The FDA's present criterion for starting zidovudine in HIV-infected infants is evidence of immunologic compromise, rather than a specific CD4 count. One might, however, base such therapy on age-appropriate CD4 values. Since counts of less than 1,500 in the first year, less than 750 in the second year, and less than 500 in years 2 through 6 indicate heightened risk of PCP and severe immunocompromise, CD4 counts somewhat higher than those values might be viewed as indicators of the need for antiviral therapy. In order to manage HIV-infected infants and children appropriately, such values would have to be carefully defined. Hypergammaglobulinemia also indicates immune compromise and may be another parameter used for initiating therapy.

The minimum CD4 levels referred to are currently used as indications for starting PCP prophylaxis (Figure 5). Their predictive value has not been substantiated by prospective studies. Rather, they are derived from retrospective evaluations of available CD4 counts in infants and children with PCP. Using these guidelines, about 90% of children who present with PCP would qualify for prophylaxis.

Although the recommended dose of zidovudine for adults has been lowered, we do not know whether that is appropriate for children. Since children have more frequent CNS involvement, they may require higher doses of zidovudine to ensure adequate drug levels in the central nervous system. The recommended dose of zidovudine for children is still 180 mg/m^2 every six hours, although that can be reduced if the child does not tolerate it well. The ACTG is currently conducting a study (protocol 128) comparing the standard dose with 90 mg/m^2 to determine whether efficacy is maintained at the reduced level and whether there is a difference in tolerance or toxicity.

Zidovudine has shown some efficacy in children. In general, the pediatric experience tends to follow the adult pattern of initial clinical improvement and prolonged survival, then waning benefits after varying intervals of time.

Additionally, zidovudine may not be consistently successful in preventing damage to all organ systems, although it is not known whether progressive disease such as cardiomyopathy is the result of virus-induced damage, an immune response made possible by drug-induced improvement in immune function, or drug toxicity. Finally, bone marrow effects from zidovudine represent the primary toxicity observed. Approximately 20% of pediatric patients already have hematologic

Figure 5. Guidelines for *Pneumocystis carinii* Pneumonia Prophylaxis in HIV-Infected Children After the First Month of Life

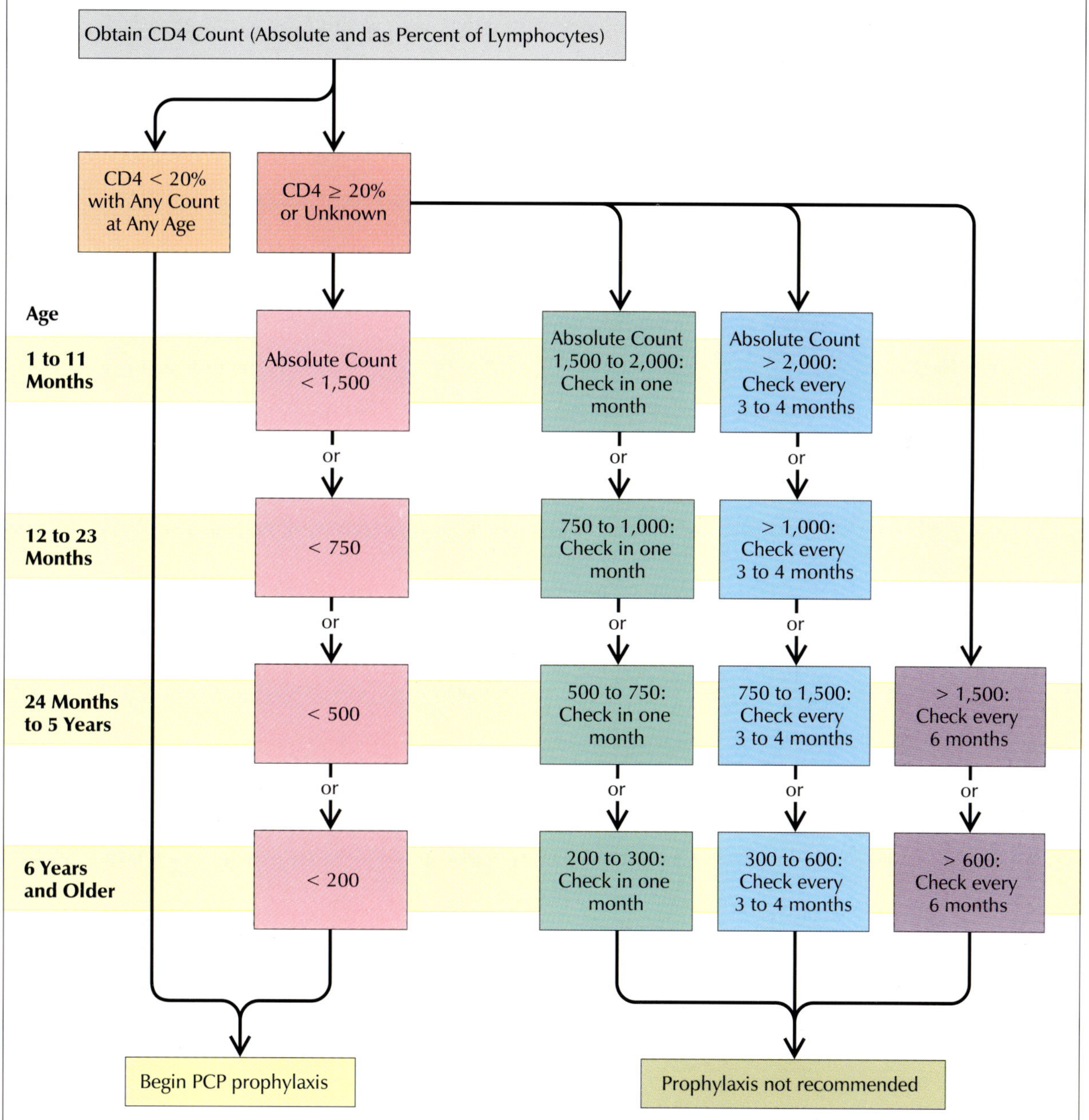

impairment from their HIV infection when they start therapy. Fortunately, zidovudine has been well tolerated by the majority of symptomatic children.

Since zidovudine alone is unlikely to offer sustained benefit for most persons with HIV infection, new antiretroviral agents are being tested, alone and in combination with zidovudine. Included are dideoxycytidine (ddC) and dideoxyinosine (ddI)—nucleoside analogues that, like zidovudine, inhibit HIV reverse transcriptase. Bone marrow stimulation with granulocyte colony-stimulating factor is under investigation as a means of counteracting bone marrow toxicity from zidovudine.

It is my opinion that every HIV-infected child should have an opportunity to be enrolled in a clinical trial. The experience with each study subject becomes part of our store of knowledge and can help in determining the most efficient way to provide medical care for all of these children.

Clinical trials can certainly become more efficient. We are trying to improve the integration of individual protocols and to develop several continuous protocols with uniform permissive inclusion criteria and standardized end points. A prototype protocol could have the appropriate standard therapy as the control arm. This plan would require fewer subjects than would separate control arms for each protocol.

In addition, researchers trying to build on earlier work need to have the flexibility to study a new drug quickly, which might be effected by opening an arm on an existing study and avoiding the delay involved in writing and obtaining approval for an entirely new protocol. The efficiency so gained is particularly important in pediatrics because of the relatively small number of HIV-infected children and the rapid progression of infection in this population.

The rapid progression of a fatal disease and the need for better therapy argue for changing the traditional mode of testing of investigational agents. Most researchers now agree that pediatric phase I trials should begin simultaneously with or only shortly after those in adults.

Treatment protocols and programs cannot focus exclusively on medication. These children are for the most part completely dependent on others. They are taken to the doctor and dependent on parents and other care providers for the necessities of daily living. A disproportionate amount of HIV infection in families involves those who are socioeconomically disadvantaged, with little access to the health care system. These patients are greatly in need of social services both to facilitate and to complement their medical care. To cite but one example from our experience, it is not appropriate to discharge a child from the hospital with a central venous line to provide nutritional support if he will be returning in wintertime to a home with no heat or hot water and no telephone.

The social problems these children face may be compounded by fear of this infection. In contrast to children with other life-threatening diseases, those with HIV infection often encounter a lack of school and community support, despite the fact that such infection has not ever been shown to be contagious in school or day-care settings.

Passive Immunization

Intravenous immune globulin, successful in children with congenital immunoglobulin deficiencies, was used early in the HIV epidemic in an attempt to diminish the risk of infections. The National Institute of Child Health and Human Development has completed a randomized placebo-controlled study of IV immune globulin in HIV-infected children. Most did not receive antiretroviral therapy, although PCP prophylaxis with co-trimoxazole (trimethoprim-sulfamethoxazole) was used as clinically indicated. There was no difference in survival. The study did demonstrate, however, a decrease in bacterial infections in children with CD4 counts greater than 200.

It is not known whether this benefit may also be seen in children receiving antiretroviral therapy. ACTG protocol 051, a placebo-controlled trial of IV immune globulin in children receiving zidovudine, is studying the question. Until its data become available, our management approach is to administer immune globulin to HIV-infected children if they are hypogammaglobulinemic or have demonstrated a susceptibility to invasive bacterial infections. We do not routinely administer IV immune globulin to symptomatic HIV-positive children.

Vaccination

HIV status should not affect a child's vaccination schedule. On the contrary, special consideration should be given to vaccines against two diseases: polio and measles.

Inactivated polio vaccine is a prudent choice for HIV-positive children and their contacts, to eliminate the risk of disease from pathogenic mutations of the vaccine virus. Live oral polio vaccine continues to be universally used in developing countries, and vaccine-related disease has yet to be reported. For the present, the risk remains strictly theoretical.

HIV-positive children do not always mount an adequate antibody response to vaccination. In particular, vaccination with attenuated measles virus may not confer protection, especially in children with symptomatic HIV infection. HIV-seropositive children should receive measles vaccine. And HIV-seropositive children who are exposed to measles should be given passive immunoglobulin prophylaxis even if they have been immunized.

HIV Infection in Adolescents

Adolescents acquire HIV infection by much the same routes as do adults. Where adolescents differ substantially from adults is in their perception of risk, which is evidenced by a lack of noticeable change in high-risk behavior. Their denial is reinforced by the long incubation period of the disease: 15-year-olds, for example, may be unimpressed by the danger of AIDS developing after age 21 because that span of years is beyond their emotional horizon. They would be more easily convinced if the long-term consequences were more apparent among their peers.

The statistics suggest that sexual activity is the most common means of HIV transmission among adolescents: homosexual activity in the case of males and heterosexual activity in the case of females. In both groups, transmission is frequently from older men who have been sexually active for a longer period. That epidemiologic pattern occurs consistently with sexually transmitted diseases, and it is one that adolescents should be made aware of. The clinical course of AIDS among adolescents, and their response to treatment, are also closer to those of adults.

The Challenges

Until we can effectively prevent vertical transmission of HIV, the scope of the AIDS epidemic in children will reflect that of HIV infection in women of childbearing age. Current trends are not encouraging. According to conservative estimates by the CDC, the death rate from HIV infection in women 15 to 44 years of age in the United States quadrupled between 1985 and 1988, while other causes of death remained stable. Mortality is particularly pronounced in the Northeast and in black women. By 1987, rates in black women in New Jersey and New York were comparable to those of women in the Ivory Coast of Africa. In that same year, AIDS was the second leading cause of death in black children one to four years old in New Jersey and New York.

Nationwide, by 1992 AIDS is projected to be among the five leading causes of death in women of childbearing age and in children one to four years old. Given that pattern, a matrix of comprehensive family-centered care and management will be essential. In addition to their medical needs, households need help coping with terminal illness—a burden that may otherwise prove insupportable, especially when more than one person in a family is infected.

Bringing an HIV-infected child into the health care system usually provides the opportunity to bring the mother into the system as well. Frequently, she will not have been aware of the availability of treatment or will have denied her need for it. Measures for circumventing denial are necessary. We have found that if mothers are advised or urged to go to a clinic, they tend not to go by themselves. The clinic for women needs to be in the same location (and open at the same time) as that for children. If someone will accompany the mothers to the clinic—literally lead them by the hand, in some cases—and provide care for their children, they will take the time to go to the clinic. Once they become accustomed to the routine, acquire confidence in their physicians, and have accepted the fact of their illness, they will participate in their own care.

Pediatric and maternal AIDS seems destined to affect large segments of our society, whether directly or indirectly. To mitigate the suffering caused by this epidemic and to curtail the epidemic's spread, it will be necessary to continue the search for effective prevention and more effective treatment, along with a greater commitment to health care for the disadvantaged.

SELECTED READING

Pizzo PA, Wilfert CM (Eds): Pediatric AIDS: The Challenge of HIV Infection in Infants, Children, and Adolescents. Williams & Wilkins, Baltimore, 1991

Centers for Disease Control: Guidelines for prophylaxis against *Pneumocystis carinii* pneumonia for children infected with human immunodeficiency virus. MMWR 40(RR-2): 1, 1991

Chu SY, Buehler JW, Berkelman RL: Impact of the human immunodeficiency virus epidemic on mortality in women of reproductive age, United States. JAMA 264: 225, 1990

European Collaborative Study: Children born to women with HIV-1 infection: Natural history and risk of transmission. Lancet 337: 253, 1991

Halsey NA et al: Transmission of HIV-1 infections from mothers to infants in Haiti: Impact on childhood mortality and malnutrition. JAMA 264: 2088, 1990

McKinney RE Jr et al: A multicenter trial of oral zidovudine in children with advanced human immunodeficiency virus disease. N Engl J Med 324: 1018, 1991

Pizzo PA et al: Effect of continuous intravenous infusion of zidovudine (AZT) in children with symptomatic HIV infection. N Engl J Med 319: 889, 1988

Auger I et al: Incubation periods for paediatric AIDS patients. Nature 336: 575, 1988

8 Reducing Occupational Risk of HIV Infection

JULIE LOUISE GERBERDING
University of California, San Francisco

It has been a decade since acquired immunodeficiency syndrome first came to the attention of medical investigators, and over seven years since the first incident of occupational transmission of human immunodeficiency virus (type 1) was reported. In the interim, protective strategies for avoiding workplace exposures to HIV and other blood-borne pathogens have been refined, and protocols for antiviral chemoprophylaxis of exposed workers are now in widespread use. Nevertheless, a climate of fear persists—sufficient, in some settings, to hamper delivery of health services to HIV-infected patients. There are also disturbing indications that young physicians and nurses have begun to shun training programs and practice opportunities in areas with high HIV case loads—typically, inner-city hospitals, where their services are vitally needed.

To some extent, caregiver concerns are justified. The virus is deadly, and the risk of acquiring it from an infected patient—although by all estimates very small—is certainly real. The sheer magnitude of the HIV pandemic (more than 1 million infected persons estimated in the United States alone, 8 million worldwide) suggests that it will be almost impossible for most health care workers to avoid contact with HIV-infected patients in the near future. AIDS transmission may have slowed among homosexual and bisexual men and transfusion recipients, but it continues to rise among other high-risk populations, such as intravenous drug users and their sexual and needle-sharing partners. Furthermore, median survival is improving as greater numbers of patients seek early drug treatment. This trend will inevitably raise the overall number of contacts between health care workers and infected patients. It will also increase the likelihood that those requiring hospitalization will have advanced symptomatic HIV infection.

Another legitimate area of concern is job discrimination. Some employers have forbidden infected health personnel from interacting directly with patients. Others have refused to permit seropositive employees to perform invasive procedures or have insisted that employees obtain informed consent before such procedures. Inevitably, these restrictions increase the reluctance of those who believe they have been exposed on the job to take advantage of testing, counseling, and chemoprophylaxis.

The recent identification of three probable cases of practitioner-to-patient transmission of HIV by a Florida dentist has exacerbated tensions by introducing the possibility of new CDC guidelines requiring mandatory HIV testing of health workers and practice restrictions. In fact, the risk of practitioner-to-patient transmission is minute and likely to be limited to a small number of procedures (e.g., blind vaginal hysterectomy and similar "by feel" manipulations) already epidemiologically associated with hepatitis-B transmission. Retrospective reviews of more than 600 surgical patients treated by HIV-infected surgeons have failed to reveal any cases of transmission. Nevertheless, development of infection control techniques to minimize the potential for percutaneous injuries during invasive procedures is essential to further reduce risks to both patients and their health care providers.

Although some caregiver concerns are justified, others are clearly exaggerated. Medicine has never been a "zero risk" profession—although to young clinicians trained in the era of broad-spectrum antibiotics and effective vaccines, it may appear so. Infection has long been recognized as a hazard of medical practice. Looked at another way, however, the risk of acquiring HIV from a patient is substantially less than that of acquiring hepatitis B or many other potentially life-threatening illnesses. More than 200 infected health care workers in the United States die each year of complications of occupationally acquired HBV, yet little concern about that is evident. Even though an effective HBV vaccine exists and its use has been widely promulgated, in many centers fewer than 40% of practitioners at risk have been immunized to date.

Of course, HBV is only *potentially* life threatening, whereas a diagnosis of HIV infection is viewed as a death sentence. The possible mutability of the virus, the current fatal course of its infection, and the lack of definitive therapies have lent HIV a stigma unrivaled by any disease of modern times—and probably by any since the Black Death of the Middle Ages. Although no transmissions have been documented during routine patient care (unless parenteral exposure occurred), fear of contagion from even casual contact with seropositive patients persists in many quarters. As a result, HIV-infected patients may receive less than optimal care. Practitioner reactions may also be colored by disapproval of the life-styles of homosexual or drug-abusing patients or by the emotional conflicts arising from care of any patient with a terminal disease.

Acknowledgment of such reactions and of the stress involved in caring for AIDS patients is an important prerequisite for proper care of such patients. Physicians and other health care personnel should evaluate their fears about occupational acquisition of HIV in light of epidemiologic evidence (which will be presented) and then determine the extent to which such fears may be unjustified. Total eradication of fear is not a realistic or even desirable goal. Instead, caregiver concerns should be acknowledged and channeled into constructive action, such as careful attention to precautions regarding exposure to patients' body fluids. Other positive goals include modification of high-risk procedures (with special attention to avoidance of needle-stick injury), postexposure chemoprophylaxis (if appropriate), and support for co-workers who have inadvertently been exposed to HIV.

Assessing Occupational Risk

The scientific data base on occupationally acquired HIV is derived from a number of different sources with varying degrees of reliability. The gold standard is represented by documented seroconversions that have been reported either in the medical literature or to health departments and the CDC. As of mid-1990, 27 documented seroconversions had been reported (Figure 1). Twenty-two of these were subsequent to needle-stick or similar percutaneous exposures.

It is generally accepted that documented seroconversions are underreported, in part because of the reluctance of exposed workers to step forward and also because not every case is considered sufficiently newsworthy or well documented to be cited. In 1990, a letter to the *New England Journal of Medicine* created a furor when the writer observed that one highly publicized case of presumed occupational HIV infection had not been included in the Public Health Service data base. The implication was that authorities had knowingly allowed a number of such cases

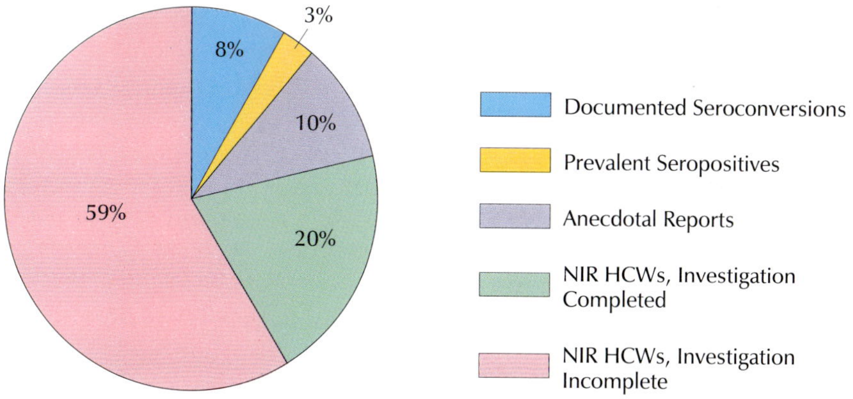

Figure 1 Among 327 case reports of health care personnel with HIV infection, there were only 27 in which diagnostic criteria met the gold standard for occupational acquisition—documented seroconversions. The rest were an amalgam of less reliable reports, most involving investigations of health care workers (HCWs) who denied life-style factors and thus had no identified risk (NIR) other than occupation.

to "slip through the cracks" in order to minimize the magnitude of risk associated with care of HIV-infected patients.

The CDC is currently implementing a cooperative program of surveillance, investigation, and reporting of cases of occupationally acquired HIV to improve estimates of the actual number of exposed workers. Cross-sectional data derived from seroprevalence studies of particular groups, such as health care personnel in the U.S. military, allow estimation of the relative risk associated with employment in a health care profession. In one grouping of 13 independent prevalence studies conducted between 1985 and 1988, 21 (0.32%) of 6,619 health care workers tested for HIV were seropositive. Estimates of the prevalence of HIV in the U.S. general population range from 0.12% to 0.80%. Thus, health care worker seroprevalence lies somewhere in the mid-range of population-based estimates.

Seroprevalence data have a number of obvious limitations. First, the timing and circumstances of exposure cannot be ascertained. Second, there is no way of confirming that HIV seropositivity is related to workplace exposures, as many caregivers also acknowledge having a community-based high-risk life-style. Third, because the rate of HIV infection in the U.S. population has been steadily increasing, prevalence studies in the mid-1980s probably do not provide an accurate reflection of HIV infection's current prevalence in the medical community.

Less helpful are reports of caregivers who have acquired AIDS but deny having a community-based high-risk life-style and have therefore been categorized as "no identified risk" (NIR). It is highly likely that many of these persons actually became infected off the job but have been reluctant to state so because of concerns about financial compensation, disclosure of sexual preference, or (in the case of intravenous drug abusers) loss of job or professional licensure. Since distinguishing between these cases and true occupational transmissions is virtually impossible, it is widely assumed that AIDS surveillance data in the NIR category tend to err on the side of exaggerating occupational risk of HIV infection.

Fourteen longitudinal studies of cohorts of health care workers involved in daily care of HIV-infected patients are currently under way. Thus far, 1,962 study participants have sustained percutaneous exposures to HIV-infected blood or blood-containing body fluids. Of these, six have manifested serologic evidence of HIV infection, an infection rate per exposed participant of 0.32% (Table 1). (In contrast, the risk of acquiring hepatitis B after needle-stick exposure is somewhere in the neighborhood of 10% to 35%. The higher transmission rate in this context is probably a reflection of the fact that HBV titers in the blood of infected patients are typically higher—by several orders of magnitude—than HIV titers.) Although a handful of anecdotal case reports documented HIV transmission through mucocutaneous exposure, the risk from cutaneous or mucous membrane contact via skin lesions has remained too low to be measured in the prospective studies despite several thousand exposures of this type.

Table 1. Occupational Risk of HIV Transmission After Percutaneous Exposure: Data from 14 Prospective Studies*

Health care workers	1,962
Percutaneous exposures	2,006
Seroconversions	6
Infection rate per worker	0.32%
Infection rate per exposure	0.31%

*All workers seronegative within 30 days of percutaneous exposure to blood or blood-containing body fluids from a patient known to be HIV infected; subsequent follow-up at least 90 days after exposure

Equal risk has been attributed to all percutaneous injuries, although logic tells us that workers who are more seriously injured or exposed to large volumes of blood or to highly viremic blood have greater cause for concern. No attempt has thus far been made to distinguish between the risk during limited exposures to HIV and that of dramatic exposures involving deep penetration, a large inoculum of blood, or highly concentrated commercial virus specimens. Furthermore, even longitudinal studies have not shed much light on the relative frequency of exposure in different populations of caregivers or on the lifetime risk of HIV associated with such populations.

Looked at in its entirety, the data base suggests that the occupational risk of HIV for all U.S. health care workers lies somewhere in the neighborhood of 0.3%. Clearly, however, risk to the *individual* worker may be considerably lower or higher, depending on the prevalence of HIV in the patient population and the frequency and nature of the caregiver's contacts with seropositive persons.

Where does the greatest danger lie? Although high viral titers also have been found in infected cerebrospinal fluid and semen, only HIV-infected blood has been implicated as a source of exposure in infections involving clinicians. Other body fluids, including saliva, tears, urine, breast milk, amniotic fluid, and vaginal secretions, may contain low titers of HIV but have not been implicated as a source of occupational infection.

In a study of 1,307 consecutive surgical procedures performed at San Francisco General Hospital, accidental exposures to infected blood occurred during 84 (6.4%) procedures (Figure 2). Twenty-two (1.7%) of these were parenteral exposures consisting of 10 suture-needle-sticks, one hollow-needle-stick, six hand lacerations, four mucous membrane exposures (splashes in the eye), and one contamination of an open skin wound. None of the needle-sticks involved actual injection of blood, and all needle-sticks and all but one of the lacerations were judged to be superficial.

Twenty-six of 32 cutaneous exposures of the hand were due to glove

Figure 2. Observed Exposures to Patient's Blood During Surgery at San Francisco General Hospital

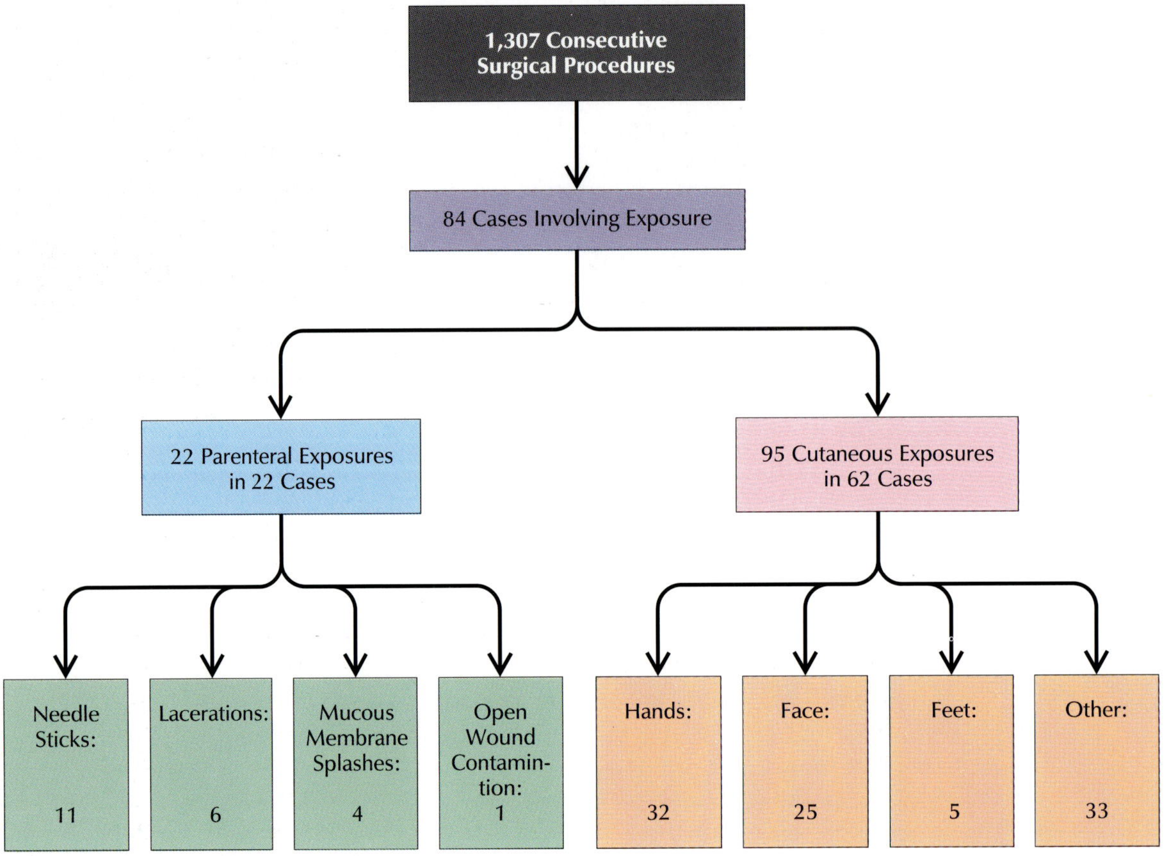

tears. Single-layer gloves were torn in 18 of these exposures, and double- or triple-layer gloves in eight. In addition, three hand exposures involved persons not wearing gloves. Goggles or glasses and masks were worn during 23 of 25 facial exposures; however, none involved workers who wore face shields. Five cutaneous foot exposures were recorded, all in personnel wearing standard, nonwaterproof surgical boots. Thirty-three cutaneous exposures at other sites were attributable to saturated clothing. Waterproof gowns were worn during only 18% of these procedures.

Neither total exposure rates nor parenteral exposure rates per 1,000 hours of surgery differed significantly among the surgical specialties, although rates in either exposure category were higher for trauma surgery, plastic surgery, obstetric and gynecologic surgery, and orthopedic surgery (Table 2). Among types of surgical personnel—attending physi-

Table 2. Exposure Rates According to Surgical Subspecialty at San Francisco General Hospital

Subspecialty	*Case Exposure Rate**	*Number of Exposures*		*Hours of Surgery*	*Exposure Rate†*	
		Total	*Parenteral*		*Total*	*Parenteral*
Trauma	9.5	25	2	322	77.6	6.2
Plastic	10.9	9	2	147	61.1	13.6
Ob/Gyn	7.4	17	4	303	56.1	13.2
Orthopedic	10.4	24	8	620	38.7	12.9
General	6.6	21	3	578	36.3	5.2
Extremity (elective)	3.7	9	2	340	26.5	5.9
Oral	6.9	2	0	78	25.6	0
Neurologic	8.3	5	0	201	24.9	0
Ear/nose/throat	1.9	4	1	239	16.7	4.2
Urologic	1.0	1	0	168	6.0	0
Minor GI procedures	0	0	0	18	0	0

*Number of cases with exposure/number of cases (%)
†Number of exposures per 1,000 hours

cians, residents, students, anesthesiologists, and nurses—surgical residents had the largest proportion of both parenteral (12 of 22) and cutaneous (41 of 95) exposures. Nurses had few parenteral exposures but sustained cutaneous hand exposures in 12 cases. Four variables were clearly associated with increased risk of exposure: major vascular procedures, intra-abdominal gynecologic surgery, procedures lasting longer than three hours, and procedures in which blood loss exceeded 300 ml.

On the basis of data obtained from this study, the theoretical occupational risk of HIV among surgical personnel at San Francisco General Hospital was calculated to be 0.125 infections per year, or one infection every eight years. It should be remembered, however, that our institution is in an area of very high HIV prevalence. There are many U.S. communities in which the theoretical occupational risk of HIV might be as low as one infection every 80 years. On the other hand, risk of exposure during cardiac and transplantation surgery was not assessed, because these procedures are not performed at this center. Since both tend to be characterized by long duration, significant blood loss, and major vascular manipulations, the occupational risk associated with these procedures may exceed our estimates.

To Test or Not to Test?

Preoperative testing for HIV has been advocated as a precautionary measure, especially in settings of high HIV prevalence. Proposals range from testing all patients scheduled for surgery to testing only those who acknowledge a high-risk life-style. Advocates of the across-the-board approach believe that preoperative testing would reduce the spread of infection by improving compliance with body fluid precautions or by promoting selective implementation of those precautions. In addition, preoperative testing would permit diagnosis of unsuspected infection in persons who might not otherwise be screened, thereby enabling them to obtain early antiviral treatment and prophylaxis against opportunistic infections.

There are, however, a number of serious problems with preoperative testing. Requiring a patient to face the psychologic and social consequences of a potentially positive test result, primarily for the benefit of care providers, is ethically questionable. To condition surgical care, or any other form of care, on a negative test result would not only be ethically improper but could incur substantial legal risk to the practitioner. In 1988, the American Medical Association Council on Ethics and Judicial Affairs clearly stated: "A physician may not ethically refuse to treat a patient whose condition is within the physician's current realm of competence solely because the patient is seropositive."

Additional considerations include the cost of HIV screening, confirmatory testing, and follow-up counseling; the possibility of a false-positive or false-negative test result; the medical institution's potential liability if confidentiality is breached; and the danger of instilling a false sense of security that could increase the odds of transmission of HBV or other blood-borne pathogens from patients judged to be HIV-negative.

Results of the previously discussed San Francisco General Hospital study do not support the use of preoperative HIV testing to enhance awareness of the risk of HIV transmission. Neither the knowledge that a given patient had been diagnosed with HIV nor the perception that another might belong to a high-risk group influenced the rate of accidental blood exposures. This was so even when the analysis included only parenteral exposures as the dependent variable.

We believe that these results have important implications for policy planning. Since 1985, staff at San Francisco General Hospital have been instructed to observe safety precautions in handling needles and other sharp instruments and to use double gloving, protective equipment, and waterproof clothing during all surgical procedures. As a result, our intraoperative blood exposure rates are thought to be comparatively low. The parenteral exposure rate in our study (1.7%) was lower than the rate (4.9%) observed by Lisa Panlilio and colleagues at Grady Memorial Hospital in Atlanta, where the prevalence of blood-borne pathogens among patients is low. These data suggest that surgical personnel who practice in areas where the prevalence of HIV is very high, such as San Francisco, are more motivated to comply with infection control precautions and are less likely to be exposed.

As long as surgical personnel maintain a high standard of infection control for all patients, little additional benefit may be expected to result from preoperative HIV testing. On the other hand, if compliance is generally poor, identifying patients, albeit expensive, may enhance safety for those cases perceived to be risky. We believe that use of procedure-specific infection control precautions, when universally employed, is a wiser course to follow and one well worth the commitment of time and effort necessary for implementation.

Infection Control Procedures

Prevention of needle-stick injury must be the highest priority in any infection control program. Approximately 100,000 accidental needlesticks are reported in the United States each year; many could be prevented by routine double gloving.

Following the observational study at San Francisco General Hospital, a validation study was conducted using the same data-collection approach in 50 randomly selected surgical procedures. All gloves worn by surgical personnel during these procedures (960 gloves) were collected, examined for visible blood contamination, punctures, or tears, and filled with water to identify occult perforations. Perforation rates (number of perforations per 100 gloves) were compared for 80 gloves worn singly, 448 double outer gloves, and 384 double inner gloves. Rates for single and double outer gloves were nearly identical—17.5% and 17.4%, respectively—and were three times higher than the rate (5.5%) for double inner gloves (Figure 3). These results are strikingly similar to those obtained in another study of glove perforation by H. Matta and co-workers in Britain, who found that double gloving resulted in an 80% reduction of inner glove perforations.

In addition to preventing needle-stick injury, double gloving provides considerable protection against cutaneous exposure to blood. In 18 of 78 cases of perforation noted in the validation study, the outer surfaces of double inner gloves were grossly contaminated with blood. We estimate that at least half of the cutaneous exposures caused by tears in single gloves might have been prevented had every staff member in the study worn an additional glove.

Although gloves are the most critical article of protective clothing recommended for health care workers exposed to blood-borne viruses, additional waterproof barriers—face shields, waterproof gowns, waterproof boots—should also be used. Among surgical personnel in the San Francisco General Hospital study, use of such barriers could have prevented more than half of observed episodes of cutaneous exposure involving sites other than the hand.

Unfortunately, not all protective garments are equally protective; 2% of the sterile surgical gloves in our study had perforations when examined immediately after removal from the package. Failure rates as high as 40% have been documented for nonsterile polyethylene examination gloves used in laboratory work with infectious agents. Obviously, these rates are much too high, and quality control by manufacturers needs to

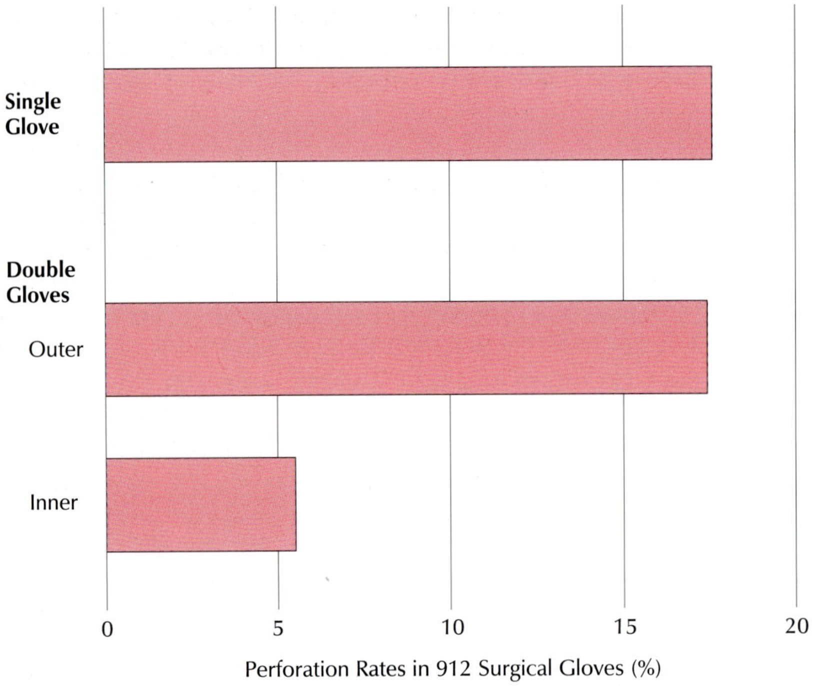

Figure 3 In the operating room, a simple and highly effective way to reduce the risk of HIV infection is double gloving, as suggested by results of a study of gloves worn by surgical personnel at San Francisco General Hospital. Perforation rates in 80 single gloves and 448 double outer gloves were virtually the same, and triple the rate in 384 double inner gloves.

be improved. Similarly, a 1990 study of surgical gowns, by Philip P. Shadduck and colleagues at Duke University, demonstrated significant differences in the ability of gown fabrics to resist penetration by HIV-containing body fluids. Seven of the 17 gown types tested failed to block HIV penetration at pressure levels found in clinical practice, and six others resisted penetration at normal levels of pressure but failed the test at higher levels. Only four types of gown fabric successfully prevented HIV penetration at all pressures.

Development of sturdier gloves and more fluid-resistant synthetic fabrics, along with such simple technical improvements as needle disposal systems, can contribute appreciably to risk reduction. But infection control procedures are only as good as the people who use them. Health care workers continue to recap needles, for example, despite the availability of puncture-resistant disposal containers. Force of habit, lack of information, and perception of competing hazards may perpetuate this unsafe behavior. Expensive new devices (such as resheathing needles) designed to be "inherently safer" represent an important advance. Testing and careful evaluation must be undertaken before they can be unconditionally recommended.

Predictably, motivation for infection control is poorest in areas where

HIV prevalence is perceived to be low. Even in areas of relatively high HIV prevalence, however, not all hospitals—and not all services within those hospitals—are equally effective in alerting personnel to the risks inherent in occupational exposures.

Universal precautions were developed by the CDC as a means of standardizing infection control and reducing patient-to-caregiver transmission of viruses and bacteria. There are five major recommendations: 1) prompt washing of hands and other skin surfaces following contact with body fluids, or immediately after gloves are removed; 2) avoidance of injury with needles, scalpels, and other sharp instruments; 3) routine use of appropriate barrier precautions; 4) avoidance of direct patient care by health care workers with skin lesions; and 5) strict adherence to infection control by pregnant health care workers, to minimize risk of perinatal transmission of blood-borne infections.

With universal precautions, the former isolation category of "blood and body fluid precautions" is eliminated. Instead, there is a minimal level of blood or body fluid isolation for all patients, irrespective of diagnosis. Further isolation precautions are added for patients with infections that are transmitted by other routes (e.g., infectious diarrhea, tuberculosis).

An alternative approach—followed at San Francisco General Hospital and many other institutions in areas of high HIV prevalence—is the system referred to as body substance precautions, or body substance isolation. In practice, these are much like the universal precautions, in that prevention of needle-stick injury and use of barrier methods of infection control are emphasized. Philosophically, however, the two are quite different. Whereas universal precautions place a clear emphasis on avoidance of blood-borne infection, body substance precautions take a more global view. The degree of contact with the blood and body fluids or tissues of each patient is considered to determine the type of precaution (if any) required. Unlike the CDC system (in which precautions are based on patient diagnosis), body substance precautions are procedure-specific, based on the degree of anticipated contact. We find that this approach is actually easier to teach and implement than universal precautions although, as noted, the end result is much the same.

Recommendations After HIV Exposure

Since June 1989, personnel at San Francisco General Hospital who believe they may have been accidentally exposed to HIV or HBV can call the "needle-stick hotline" for immediate, confidential assistance (Figure 4). The hotline, which is run by our Occupational Infectious Diseases Service, operates 24 hours a day, seven days a week. When a health care worker calls, he or she is given immediate counseling by a physician or nurse-practitioner and offered a range of services: rapid access to zidovudine therapy (if warranted); consultation with a licensed counselor;

OCCUPATIONAL INFECTIOUS DISEASES PROGRAM
A JOINT PROGRAM OF THE SFGH HIV PREVENTION SERVICE
AND THE SAN FRANCISCO DEPARTMENT OF PUBLIC HEALTH

AFTER A NEEDLESTICK, SPLASH, OR OTHER BODY FLUID EXPOSURE...

STEP 1: DECONTAMINATE
SKIN: WASH WITH SOAP AND WATER
EYES, NOSE, MOUTH: RINSE WITH WATER / SALINE

STEP 2: CALL NEEDLESTICK HOTLINE
24 HOURS EVERY DAY

STEP 3: EMPLOYEE HEALTH FOLLOW-UP

PRIMARY PREVENTION SERVICES:

* HEPATITIS SCREENING / IMMUNIZATION
* OTHER IMMUNIZATION UPDATE
* WORK SITE ASSESSMENT
* EXPOSURE SURVEILLANCE

POST-EXPOSURE SERVICES:

* NEEDLESTICK HOTLINE
* EXPERT ADVICE AND TRIAGE
* POST-EXPOSURE HIV / HEPATITIS CARE
* CONFIDENTIAL COUNSELING, TESTING AND DOCUMENTATION
* SOURCE PATIENT EVALUATION

Figure 4 At San Francisco General Hospital, personnel who may have been exposed to HIV can get immediate, confidential assistance via a hotline.

HIV and HBV testing; and standing follow-up appointments at the employee health clinic (details of the exposure are not disclosed to other hospital personnel).

The availability of counseling, support, and treatment in an atmosphere of total confidentiality has dramatically reduced barriers to reporting at our institution. Before the establishment of the hotline, surveys indicated that fewer than 30% of accidental exposures were reported to the employee health service. Reasons given for not reporting included inconvenience, not expecting any benefit (e.g., antiviral therapy), and concerns about confidentiality. In the first year of the hotline's existence, 301 occupational exposures were self-reported, as compared with only 178 the previous year (an increase of 169%). Twelve of these persons were subsequently shown to have been exposed to HIV-contaminated blood.

A month-long course of experimental zidovudine therapy was offered to all workers who reported punctures, similar injuries, or mucocutaneous exposures. In the first year, approximately 20% of HIV-exposed persons elected to begin chemoprophylaxis. Twenty of those originally started on zidovudine stopped taking the drug when informed that the source of the exposure had tested negative for HIV.

Health care workers receiving zidovudine may experience adverse side effects, the most common being nausea and fatigue. Occasionally, myalgia, headache, and fever and chills are reported. Relative neutropenia has been seen in heath care workers taking zidovudine for more than one week, although drops in absolute neutrophil counts have not been observed at San Francisco General Hospital. Neutropenia resolves quickly after discontinuance of therapy. (Both neutropenia and relative anemia have been documented with longer courses of zidovudine in immunosuppressed patients.)

Our current protocol for zidovudine prophylaxis is outlined in Table 3. As soon as possible after exposure—preferably, within the first hour—the health care workers who verbally consent to participate in the chemoprophylaxis protocol are sent to the hospital pharmacy, where a starter pack is available on request. No identification or prescription is required. (If the worker decides to continue drug treatment, written consent is obtained through the employee health service.) Meanwhile, HIV testing is arranged, details of the incident are recorded in a confidential record-keeping system, and arrangements are made for counseling and long-term follow-up. Consent is also obtained for testing the source patient.

The San Francisco General Hospital system for estimating exposure severity classifies exposures as “massive” (transfusions, parenteral exposures to HIV concentrates); “definite parenteral” (intramuscular parenteral inoculations or injections of blood or body fluids); “possible parenteral” (subcutaneous or superficial percutaneous exposures, mucous membrane splashes, contamination of open wounds); “doubtful parenteral” (exposures involving nonbloody body fluids such as saliva, urine, or tears); and “nonparenteral” (contamination of normal skin). Chemoprophylaxis is not offered to care providers in the last category. In all other categories, the decision is left to the exposed care provider, although we encourage persons in the “massive” and “definite parenteral” categories to give the possibility serious consideration. Recommended zidovudine dosages are 200 mg every four hours on days 1 through 3, followed by 100 to 200 mg every four hours for the remainder of the 28-day cycle.

Thus far, risk of severe acute toxicity with short periods of zidovudine treatment appears to be slight, particularly in a population of otherwise healthy adults. It should be emphasized, however, that the full range of long-term side effects associated with this class of drugs is still unknown. All patients in our treatment program are closely monitored for signs of hematologic, hepatic, renal, or neurologic dysfunction. Because safety in pregnancy has not been established, pregnant women are advised to avoid chemoprophylaxis unless exposure is severe. Others of childbearing age are advised to use barrier contraceptive methods and avoid conception during treatment and two weeks afterward.

When we discuss protocols for chemoprophylaxis, it is with the caveat that these are unproven therapies. We do not have enough information about the biology of early HIV infection to know whether zidovudine, or any of the current candidate antiretroviral agents, can suppress viral replication in target cells. The animal data have been inconsistent: Studies with feline and murine retrovirus models have shown suppression of viremia when zidovudine was administered shortly after viral inoculation. In SCID (severe combined immunodeficiency) mice receiving high titers of HIV, appearance of the virus was delayed but not completely attenuated even when chemoprophylaxis was begun 24 hours before inoculation.

Data from primates injected with simian immunodeficiency virus have been even more discouraging; in three studies, viral replication was not adequately prevented even when treatment was begun eight hours or, in one case, 24 hours before inoculation. Of course, these animals were exposed to extremely high titers of HIV, introduced by the intravenous rather than the transcutaneous route.

Three reported cases of postexposure zidovudine failure have similarly involved very dramatic exposures, delayed treatment, or the possibility of zidovudine-resistant viruses. Although these reports are discouraging, they may not be relevant to the vast majority of accidental exposures. At this writing, none of the exposed personnel who received anti-HIV prophylaxis through the San Francisco General Hospital program has become infected. Whether this is luck or a direct result of pharmacologic intervention remains to be seen.

The counseling component of our postexposure protocol was initially conceived as an adjunct to the drug therapy component. However, the reverse has turned out to be the case. A supportive environment and discussion of the stresses of viral exposure with a mental health professional have proved to be the most valuable aspects of our program. Among the issues addressed are the relative degree of infection risk associated with a particular exposure, symptoms of early HIV infection, protection of confidentiality, economic concerns, community resources available to exposed workers, reactions of family members, and use of safer sexual practices until infection has been ruled out. Family members or sexual partners are frequently included in the counseling process.

To the caregiver who has been accidentally exposed to HIV, the risk of seroconversion does not feel like 0.4% but more like 400%. Management decisions should therefore be predicated not only on a realistic assessment of the scientific data base but also on appreciation of the concerns of those directly affected by occupational exposure. Just as physicians and other health professionals have an ethical obligation to care for HIV-infected patients, medical institutions have a responsibility to implement risk reduction strategies and provide economic security and psychosocial support for those in whom the infection results from occupational exposure.

SELECTED READING

Beekmann SE et al: Risky business: Using necessarily imprecise casualty counts to estimate occupational risks for HIV-1 infection. Infect Control Hosp Epidemiol 11:371, 1990

Update: Acquired immunodeficiency syndrome and human immunodeficiency virus infection among health care workers. MMWR 37:229, 1988

Kelley PW et al: Human immunodeficiency virus seropositivity among members of the active duty US Army 1985–89. Am J Public Health 80:405, 1990

Cowan D et al: Prevalence of HIV infection among persons employed in medicine and health occupations. Presented at the Fifth International Conference on AIDS, Montreal, Quebec, 1989

Gerberding JL, Henderson DK: Design of rational infection control guidelines for human immunodeficiency virus infection. J Infect Dis 156:861, 1987

Henderson DK, Gerberding JL: Prophylactic zidovudine after occupational exposure to the human immunodeficiency virus type-1: An interim analysis. J Infect Dis 160:321, 1989

Position paper: The HIV-infected healthcare worker. Infect Control Hosp Epidemiol 11:647, 1990

Gerberding JL et al: Risk of exposure of surgical personnel to patients' blood during surgery at San Francisco General Hospital. N Engl J Med 322:1788, 1990

Panlilio AL et al: Blood contacts during surgical procedures. JAMA 265:1533, 1991

Gerberding JL, Schecter WP: Surgery and AIDS: Reducing the risk (editorial). JAMA 265:1572, 1991

9 Partner Notification for HIV Control

FRANKLYN N. JUDSON *Denver Public Health*

Partner notification, formerly known as "contact tracing," refers to efforts by infected persons or health care providers to notify those who may have been exposed to a communicable pathogen—in this case, human immunodeficiency virus. For decades, public health agencies in this country have successfully used partner notification to control sexually transmitted diseases. Because HIV is spread primarily among sex or needle-sharing partners, it would seem to be a logical target for the basic components of partner notification programs—namely, informing those who have been exposed and offering testing, counseling, and, when appropriate, drug therapy. In many public health jurisdictions, this has not happened. The reasons include concerns about the consequences of potential breaches of confidentiality in HIV partner notification programs, the cost-effectiveness of such programs, and the efficacy of available treatment for those so identified.

In some states with large numbers of HIV infections, legislative measures have been drafted meticulously to protect the privacy of those infected. California, for example, has specifically prohibited confidential reporting of new HIV infections by patient name. In effect, this has discouraged exchange of HIV test results among health care providers and notification of exposed persons by public health professionals. The potentially high cost of locating and testing HIV case contacts in a city such as San Francisco is the most frequently cited explanation for not instituting such measures.

In New York, state law provides for confidential HIV testing but also includes the option of anonymous testing. Although a statute effective February 1, 1989, gave New York physicians permission to notify partners of seropositive patients or refer their names to the state health department, most have been reluctant to become involved. As former New York City Health Commissioner Stephen C. Joseph (an outspoken advocate of HIV testing and partner notification) has pointed out, "permission to warn" does not carry the same ethical, medical, or legal imperative as "duty to warn."

The Colorado Approach

The state of Colorado has taken a different approach to partner notification as a public health tool for HIV control. In the fall of 1985—within eight months of FDA approval of the enzyme-linked immunosorbent assay (ELISA) for HIV antibody—the Colorado State Board of Health voted unanimously to amend the state's communicable disease reporting regulations. Positive ELISA and Western blot antibody tests and virus cultures were added to the list of results automatically reported by clinical laboratories to state and local health departments. Results were recorded by patient name, to permit accurate tracking of infection and allow responsible health care agencies to recall HIV-positive patients for counseling and evaluation for treatment options, including antiviral therapy and *Pneumocystis carinii* prophylaxis. However, proof of identification was not required, and use of pseudonyms, particularly by homosexual men, can be common, resulting in a de facto anonymous testing option.

All information was to be held in strictest confidence and could not be released to insurance companies, employers, or other parties—not even with the specific written consent of the person tested. (In fairness, it should be pointed out that, unlike some states, Colorado has no antisodomy law. Thus, while a hypothetical breach of confidentiality might subject an HIV-positive person to psychological damage or job discrimination, it could not result in prosecution for illegal sex acts.)

With the support of public health officials, a subsequent Colorado statute, passed in 1987, further strengthened the confidentiality provisions of HIV-reporting regulations by specifying that test results could not be made public "upon subpoena, search warrant, discovery proceedings, or otherwise...." The bill also superseded a 1947 quarantine statute, designed to isolate persons who refused to cooperate with statewide disease-control efforts, by incorporating rights to due process, appeals, and confidentiality. The present measure, which was strongly supported by Colorado public health officials, requires that all reasonable efforts be made to obtain the individual's voluntary cooperation; that the burden of proof be on the Department of Health to show by "clear and convincing evidence" that restrictive actions are justified in the case in question; that actions against recalcitrant persons be taken only to the extent necessary to protect the public health; that the individual may appeal any health department order in court; and that such court hearings and their transcripts or records be kept closed and confidential.

During the debate over the HIV/AIDS bill and immediately following its passage, certain segments of the homosexual community waged a heated campaign in favor of complete anonymity rather than strict confidentiality of test results. They were backed by local representatives of the American Civil Liberties Union, which opposes name reportability of HIV infections in any form. Some even called for a boycott of Department of Health testing and counseling centers and for establishment of underground testing. That this advice has not generally been heeded is evident from the observation that by 1990 an estimated 75% of the state's male homosexual population had already received publicly supported voluntary HIV testing and counseling.

Confidential vs Anonymous

A comparison of Colorado's testing statistics with those of California, which, as noted, does not allow name reportability, is instructive. During the two-year period covered in Figure 1, curves for testing activity in the two states were virtually superimposable. Apparently, whatever factors influenced test-seeking behavior operated more or less equally in each state. Neither implementation of compulsory laboratory reporting of HIV test results in 1985 nor passage of the AIDS control bill that followed seems to have deterred concerned Coloradans from seeking testing and counseling. On the contrary, during the period in question, Colorado

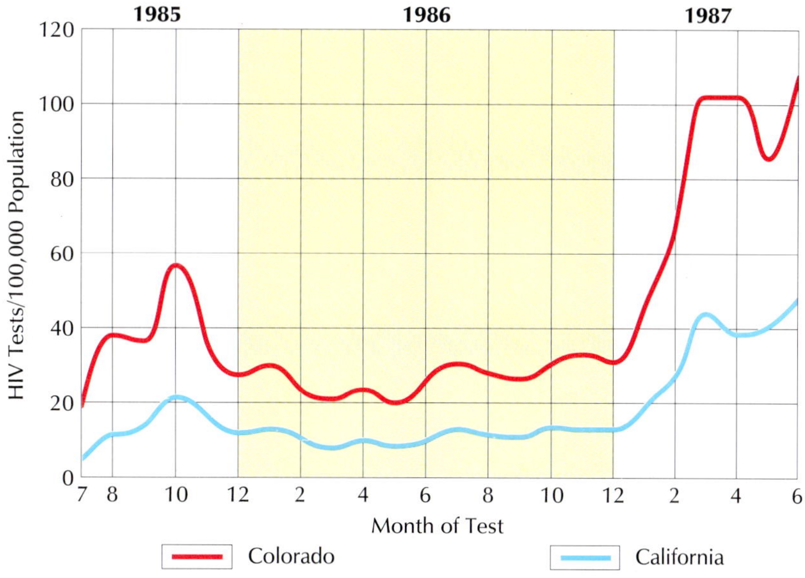

Figure 1 From July 1985 through June 1987, public programs for HIV testing in Colorado and California had closely parallel activity levels. This period includes the first several months following Colorado's adoption of confidential reporting of test results by name, which contrasts with California's requirement of strictly anonymous testing. The curves suggest that name reporting had no adverse effect on HIV-testing activity. On the contrary, throughout the two-year period the rates at which name-reportable Coloradans were tested in public programs remained consistently higher than those for anonymous Californians.

provided 41% more voluntary HIV tests per 100,000 population than did California.

Another comparison, involving Colorado and Oregon, is also informative. In December 1986, Oregon switched from exclusively confidential HIV testing to a system that offered the option of anonymous testing. Recently, Richard E. Hoffman and co-workers at the Colorado Department of Health analyzed Oregon and Colorado testing data for 1987 and 1988. They used mid-1987 population estimates in each state to deduce and compare testing and seropositivity rates according to gender, sexual orientation, and intravenous drug use.

The investigators found that among homosexual men, the testing rate in Colorado was apparently higher (estimated $p<0.05$) than that in Oregon. Colorado testing rates for all persons, all men, and women were also higher (Table 1). In addition, Colorado seropositivity rates in women and IV drug users were higher, and there was not significant difference between the two states in other categories.

Among other points, these data indicate that name reportability has not been a significant deterrent to HIV testing in Colorado. What it *has*

Table 1. Number of HIV Tests and Estimated Testing Rates in Colorado vs Oregon, 1987–88

Population Group	*Colorado*		*Oregon*	
	Tests	*Rate**	*Tests*	*Rate**
All subjects	24,377	739.5	16,184†	601.6
Men	14,199	866.0	9,084	688.6
Women	10,178	614.4	6,974	508.7
Homosexual men	5,100	5,100.0	3,792	4,710.6
IV drug users	3,133	95.1	2,511	93.4

*Per 100,000 of state population †Sex not reported in 126

done is to permit 1) more accurate tracking of the course of the epidemic in the state; 2) more effective notification, testing, counseling, and health care referral of exposed partners; and 3) systematic follow-up of the 10% to 15% of persons who fail to report for counseling after testing positive for HIV. Furthermore, as new therapies become available, the existence of personal identifier and locating information can speed up recall of persons who would benefit from antiviral treatment or administration of anti-HIV vaccines (when available), and also help to evaluate program outcomes (Table 2).

It is difficult to conceive of controlling any communicable disease without first knowing who in the population is infected or has been exposed to infection. As the scope of the epidemic broadens and many

Table 2. Advantages of Name Reportability of HIV Infection

Permits:	• More accurate estimation of prevalence • Partner notification, testing, and counseling • Follow-up of HIV-positive persons who fail to return for counseling	**May also facilitate:**	• Recalls of appropriate candidates for antiviral drugs or vaccines • Evaluation of therapeutic outcomes

persons undergo repeat testing—often under different names or at different test sites—unvalidated seroprevalence rates based on anonymous (or pseudonymous) HIV test results become increasingly difficult to interpret. Only a secure computerized records system capable of tracking test results by name and address or other identifying data can provide accurate, group-specific estimates of seropositivity prevalence and incidence.

As for trying to anticipate future health care needs on the basis of the number of patients already stricken with full-blown AIDS, an apt analogy would be trying to steer a high-speed car using only the rear-view mirror. AIDS symptoms are often not manifested until many years after seroconversion, and the ratio of asymptomatic HIV infections to AIDS cases now ranges widely from 30 to one to 10 to one or less, depending on rates of new infections.

HIV Partner Notification Strategies

Once a confidential public health records system is in place, it becomes possible discreetly to notify persons who may have been exposed unwittingly to HIV and to arrange testing and counseling for those who request it. The Centers for Disease Control has recommended that "persons who are HIV-antibody positive should be instructed in how to notify their partners and to refer them for counseling and testing. If they are unwilling to notify their partners or if it cannot be assured that their partners will seek counseling, physicians or health department personnel should use confidential procedures to assure that the partners are notified" (MMWR 37:393, 1988).

The partner notification process has been an integral part of the control of sexually transmitted diseases in the United States for nearly half a century. In such programs, data are routinely collected by state and local health departments on patients presenting with syphilis and other STDs—especially, in recent years, penicillin-resistant strains of *Neisseria gonorrhoeae*. These data are not limited to the patient's name, address, and telephone number but may include sexual preference, number of partners over a reasonable period of exposure, and whether they have been successfully contacted and referred to an STD clinic or private physician for diagnosis, counseling, and treatment. Adequacy of treatment is assessed by clinical follow-up. Although absolute privacy cannot exist in the context of a medical registry, patient confidentiality is very tightly guarded. I know of no case in Colorado in which information damaging to a patient was released during a public health investigation.

When the partner notification model is applied to HIV infection, realistic goals must be set. Because the period between initial infection and clinical disease may extend for a decade or more, some persons will be unable to recall all, or even the majority, of their sexual or needle-sharing contacts. It would be futile, for example, to attempt to trace all of the anonymous sex partners of a man who had frequented the gay bathhouse scene for years. On the other hand, the same man might also have one or more regular lovers, or even a wife or girlfriend who was unaware of his high-risk behavior. Contacting such persons could save lives as well as prevent further spread of infection—including transmission to the unborn.

Patient vs provider referral. There are two basic partner notification strategies: patient referral and provider referral (Table 3). With the former, HIV-infected patients contact their partners directly and inform them of the possibility of disease transmission, encouraging them to seek testing and counseling. A health department disease intervention specialist, physician, or other health care provider may advise the patient on what to say and how to say it, but responsibility for contacting partners rests solely with the patient.

Obviously, this is the less costly approach inasmuch as few professional resources are required, but patient referral has certain basic limitations:

Table 3. Partner Notification Strategies: Patient vs Provider Referral

	Advantages	*Disadvantages*
Patient referral	Low cost	No assurance that contacts are reached No control over quality of information delivered Automatic loss of confidentiality
Provider referral	Confidentiality protected Greater likelihood of reaching contacts Control over quality of information delivered	High cost

• First, it is impossible to ensure that all of the patient's partners have been notified or that the information they have received is accurate. In a study presented at the Fourth International Conference on AIDS (1988), A. E. Williams and co-workers of the American Red Cross Collaborative Study Group reported that six to 12 months after notification of HIV seropositivity, only 65 of 101 blood donors had revealed their test results to even their primary sexual contacts. Given the difficulty of changing established patterns of sexual activity or substance abuse, and the immense heterogeneity of human behavior in general, it would be foolhardy to assume that patients will always act out of concern for either their own health or the health of others.

• Second, patient referral inevitably reveals the identity of the HIV source. For many seropositive persons, the knowledge that they will have to face a partner directly—particularly if that partner had been unaware of the patient's sexual or drug habits—presents a formidable barrier to notification. In addition, the patient may fear that once the contact has been informed, word could leak out to others and result in discriminatory actions or, in the case of an IV drug user, the possibility of arrest for drug possession.

With provider referral, partners are never informed of the identity of the index patient or told when the alleged exposure occurred. Notification and counseling are usually performed by highly trained health department disease intervention specialists from the partner's home jurisdiction. Although this approach is more costly, it has the advantage of assuring that high-quality information reaches the exposed person in a manner likely to be understood. Nevertheless, since responsibility for naming sex or needle-sharing partners still resides with the patient, the best efforts of caregivers and public health workers can occasionally be frustrated by a patient who will not cooperate.

Rationale

Critics of HIV partner notification programs often cite the number of contacts missed as justification for abandoning the effort. In my view, this misses the point. In any STD control project, individual patients will be unwilling or unable to identify a certain percentage of their contacts. What is remarkable—as demonstrated by experience in Colorado and elsewhere—is the number of persons exposed to HIV infection who *are* located in the course of a properly administered health department investigation.

Furthermore, because the groups at highest risk for HIV are relatively small, their sexual or drug-using interactions tend to overlap. For example, Randolph F. Wykoff and co-workers at the South Carolina Department of Health and Environmental Control reported (JAMA 259:3563, 1988) that investigation of one HIV-positive man and his 19 sex partners resulted in the identification of a total of 90 sexual contacts. Of these, 68 were tested and 12 were found to be HIV-positive

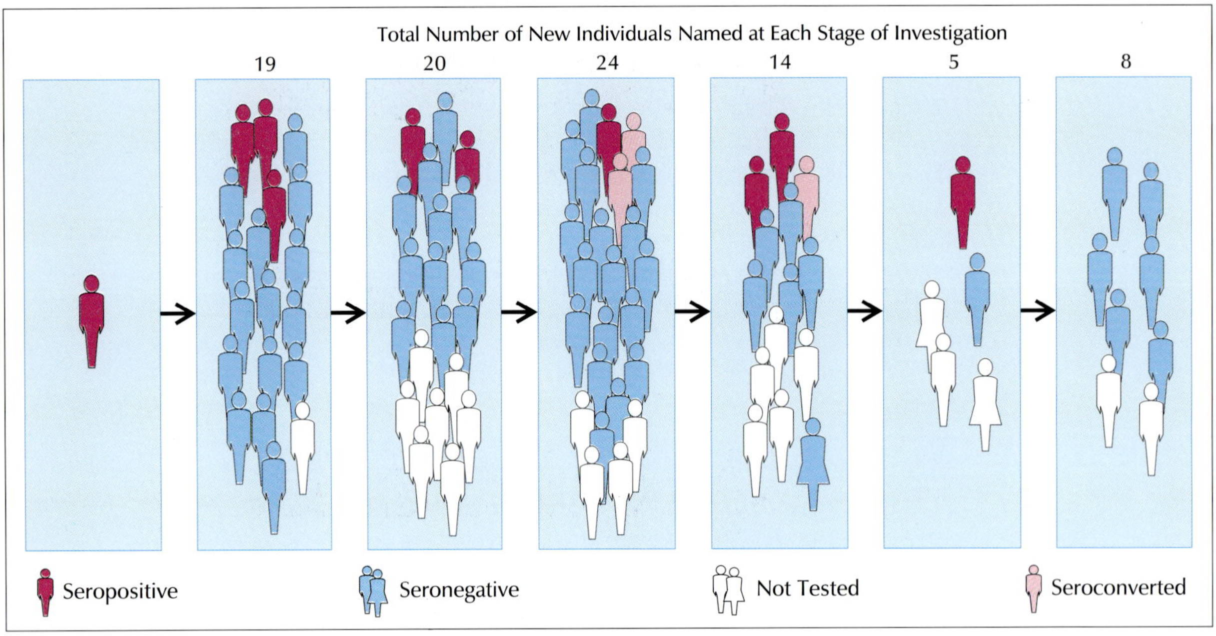

Figure 2 Partner notification programs can be highly productive, as illustrated by results of a South Carolina investigation that began with one HIV-positive man. Of the 19 sexual contacts he named, all but one were tested, and three were seropositive. Those three then named 20 sexual contacts not already identified, leading to discovery of two more HIV-positive men, who in turn named 24 other previously unidentified contacts, and so forth. When the investigation reached its end point of no new HIV-positive contacts, it had identified a total of 90 persons at risk, tested 68 of them, and found 12 who either were seropositive or seroconverted six months after initial testing.

(Figure 2). In this investigation, the 90 identified contacts were named 159 times. As John J. Potterat and colleagues at the El Paso County Health Department, Colorado Springs, and the Colorado Department of Health, Denver, have observed, such findings illustrate how productive partner notification programs can be. If one patient refuses to identify a given partner, two other patients may willingly do so. Potterat and co-workers have also noted that this is a recurring pattern in gonorrhea epidemiology.

Another argument against HIV partner notification relates to our inability to offer curative medical treatment. "Why bother spending taxpayer dollars to identify potential victims of a disease for which pharmacologic interventions are futile and no effective vaccine exists?" The answer, of couse, is that while HIV infection is certainly lethal, many of its manifestations are already treatable, and the standard of medical care is moving rapidly toward earlier treatment of asymptomatic infections.

In a prospective study of 4,323 AIDS cases reported to the San Francisco Department of Public Health between July 1981 and December 31, 1987, George F. Lemp and colleagues found significantly improved survival among patients with or without *P. carinii* pneumonia diagnosed with AIDS in 1986 and 1987 who received zidovudine, compared with

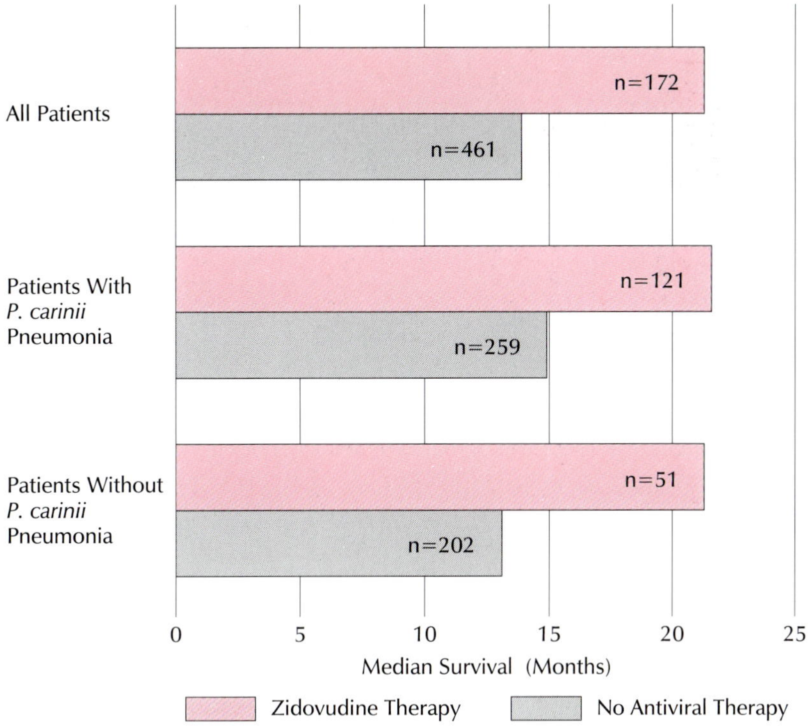

Figure 3 Among 633 patients diagnosed with AIDS in 1986–87, those treated with zidovudine had significantly improved actuarially predicted survival compared with those who received no antiviral therapy. The survival advantage for treated patients included those with or without *Pneumocystis carinii* pneumonia at or within three months of AIDS diagnosis.

those who did not receive any antiviral therapy (Figure 3). These findings support the results of earlier studies that documented increased survival of HIV patients who received zidovudine. Agents specifically directed against *P. carinii*, which threatens the lives of more that two thirds of patients with AIDS, also improve survival; these agents include aerosolized pentamidine and co-trimoxazole.

Thus initiation of appropriate pharmacotherapy in seropositive partners of patients who have tested positive for HIV may indeed prolong life. Furthermore, in states that have instituted computerized HIV registries, seropositive partners can be recalled for further treatment as new agents are approved, and seronegative partners can be notified promptly of the development of protective vaccines.

Even if effective medical treatment for AIDS symptomatology did not exist, the educational component of HIV partner notification programs would provide sufficient justification for their existence. Through targeted and individualized risk reduction counseling, the provider referral strategy of partner notification attempts to effect safer sexual behavior by personalizing risk. Within the homosexual community, personal counseling about safer sex has repeatedly been shown to alter behavior. As for

IV drug users, use of sterile "works" (needles, syringes, mixers, etc) will undoubtedly help to reduce HIV transmission. The extent of the reduction, however, would be difficult to gauge.

In dealing with HIV, any method that is acceptable to the target population and contributes to interruption of disease transmission should be utilized. It is significant that among the minority of Colorado HIV contacts who refused testing, virtually all accepted counseling offers. Similar results have been obtained elsewhere in this country and in Scandinavia.

Partner Notification in Colorado

When the state of Colorado had both the serologic and the statutory tools (including strong confidentiality protections) needed for an effective partner notification program, it assumed the ethical, medical, and legal obligations to inform persons exposed to HIV of their risk and to provide confidential testing and counseling for those willing to accept such services. This task is carried out by the STD/AIDS Section of the Colorado Department of Health and some local health departments, including the Disease Control Service of Denver Public Health (Denver Department of Health and Hospitals). The latter has performed more than half of all publicly supported HIV testing and counseling in the state, and also provided direct care to more than 30% of Colorado's AIDS patients and medical consultation to an additional 20%.

How effective have the collaborative efforts of these agencies been, and what are the implications for partner notification nationwide?

Regarding the first question, Thomas M. Vernon, executive director of the Colorado Department of Health, has noted that the initial results of partner notification in the state have been encouraging. The first 504 HIV-positive persons interviewed named 768 at-risk partners, of whom 641 were located and counseled. Tests had already been performed in 189 (72 with a positive result, 117 with a negative one). The remaining 452 persons were tested for the first time, and 68 (15%) were found to be HIV-positive (Figure 4). This positivity rate is comparable to those reported in other series.

Using these results, and making certain assumptions, Vernon has also provided an estimate of cost vs benefit in the Colorado experience with partner notification.

The assumptions were that 1) each interview and investigation sequence costs $200; 2) the estimated lifetime direct medical cost of an AIDS case not prevented is $50,000; and 3) one HIV-positive case is prevented for every two newly tested and counseled HIV-positive persons. It should be noted that the interview-investigation cost was deliberately estimated on the high side. Conversely, the estimate for the frequency of infection in the absence of intervention was quite conservative.

On this basis, Vernon concluded that effective behavior-modifying counseling of the 68 newly identified infected persons would prevent 34

Figure 4. Partner Notification in Colorado: Initial Results

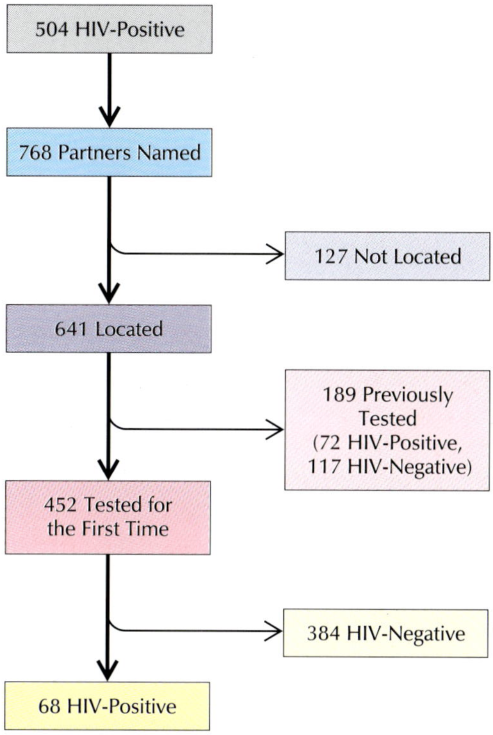

HIV infections. One could add that if the infections in only two of these persons would have progressed to AIDS, the cost of investigating some 500 index patients at $200 each would still be offset.

As for the feasibility of a nationwide effort of partner notification for HIV control, there is an obvious yardstick for comparison: this country's programs for controlling other STDs. Potterat and co-workers have concluded that those routinely carried out programs represent a caseload far outweighing that estimated for HIV. They point out that for gonorrhea alone, the annual number of cases investigated by health department workers in all states is about 360,000. In contrast, the number of new cases of HIV in the United States currently appears to be on the order of 65,000 per year. And although HIV control programs are admittedly more time-consuming, they are no more complicated than existing STD programs and use similar resources.

Based on the Colorado experience, Potterat and colleagues have calculated the national cost of partner notification for HIV control. They estimate that one worker can manage 140 cases per year. Nationally, that means 464 workers and a total annual cost of approximately $13.5 million for incident cases of HIV infection. If such a program uncovers an additional 10,000 new cases each year, the cost might approach $16 million. Either figure would represent a small price to pay for HIV control.

In the United States today, partner notification in one form or another is required of local and state health departments as a condition for receiving federal HIV prevention dollars. As a result, all 50 states make some effort at patient referral. Unfortunately, only 22 emphasize provider referral. Among other industrialized countries, similar choices have been made at the national level. Belgium, Norway, and Sweden, for example, emphasize provider referral, whereas Canada, the United Kingdom, and Holland emphasize patient referral.

To be sure, there are certain factors that may cause any partner notification program to fall short of its potential, whether it uses the provider referral mechanism or not. Lack of awareness (or refusal to accept) that a partner may be HIV-positive, ignorance of the medical advantages of early intervention, dread of a positive test result, and, to a much lesser extent, fear of discrimination are powerful forces militating against voluntary testing. Meanwhile, potentially beneficial antiviral agents sit on the shelf; a recent investigation indicated that only a fraction of the hundreds of thousands of persons who would be medically eligible for zidovudine prophylaxis are currently receiving the drug.

Given the excellent track record of public health departments throughout the county in maintaining the confidentiality of patients who have tested positive for HIV and other STDs, and the high acceptance and favorable cost-benefit profile of partner notification programs, I strongly recommend that anonymous HIV testing be abandoned and that confidential partner notification, testing, and counseling services be routinely offered to HIV-infected persons. It is time to fully accept HIV infection within the mainstream of modern public health and medical practices.

HIV infection is already a treatable disease and may become a curable one. Intensive efforts by state public health departments to identify, test, and counsel the sex and needle-sharing partners of known HIV-infected persons are ethically and medically desirable. When appropriately managed, they pose no threat to patient confidentiality. Recent experience in Colorado has suggested that they are also cost-effective.

In view of the number of lives already lost to HIV and the burden placed on our health care resources at every level, the need for greater emphasis on basic preventive measures, such as universal confidential reporting of HIV infections and partner notification, should be self-evident.

SELECTED READING

Toomey KE, Cates W Jr: Partner notification for the prevention of HIV infection. AIDS 3(suppl 1): S57, 1989

Potterat JJ et al: Partner notification in the control of human immunodeficiency virus infection. Am J Public Health 79: 874, 1989

Judson FN: What do we really know about AIDS control? *Ibid:* 878

Hart G et al: Evaluation of sexually transmitted disease control programs in industrialized countries. *In* Sexually Transmitted Diseases, 2nd ed, Holmes KK et al (Eds). McGraw-Hill, New York, 1990, pp 1031–1040

Rothenberg RB, Potterat JJ: Strategies for management of sex partners. *Ibid*, pp 1081–1086

Ramstedt KM et al: Serologic classification and contact-tracing in the control of microepidemics of β-lactamase-producing *Neisseria gonorrhoeae*. Sex Transm Dis 12 : 209, 1985

Wigfield AS: Twenty-seven years of uninterrupted contact tracing: The "Tyneside Scheme." Br J Vener Dis 48 : 37, 1972

Centers for Disease Control: Partner notification for preventing human immunodeficiency virus (HIV) infection: Colorado, Idaho, South Carolina, Virginia. MMWR 37 : 393, 401, 1988

10 AIDS, Activism, and Ethics

DAVID J. ROTHMAN *and* HAROLD EDGAR
Columbia University

In the turbulent world of acquired immune deficiency syndrome, advocates in the AIDS community are insisting that the deadly nature of this disease should change the rules to allow more patients earlier access to new therapies. Through their advocacy, the process of drug evaluation and approval has become a means of treatment as well as research. The AIDS epidemic has effectively challenged a regulatory system derived from time-honored protocols for scientific experimentation, a system strongly reinforced by scandals and disasters in the testing and introduction of new drugs a quarter century ago.

The transforming moment in the history of drug regulation had come in 1962. Senator Estes Kefauver was winding up a lengthy and modestly successful campaign to regulate drug prices by making his case for excess pharmaceutical company profitability, even allowing for investment in new drug research and development. Then the thalidomide story broke into the headlines. This drug, widely prescribed in Europe, was being evaluated by the U.S. Food and Drug Administration. One FDA official, Frances Kelsey, concerned by reports of peripheral neuropathy, held up approval long enough for the link between thalidomide and birth defects to become known.

Although major catastrophe had been averted, some 20,000 Americans—including 3,750 women of childbearing age and 625 reported as pregnant—had already taken thalidomide on an experimental basis. In this climate, Senator Kefauver clinched his argument for stronger drug regulation. His proposed legislation passed both the House and Senate by unanimous vote.

As a result, the FDA's drug approval procedures were changed from premarket notification to premarket approval. Before 1962, new drugs could be marketed once the pharmaceutical sponsor submitted safety data, unless the FDA had reviewed the data and found them unacceptable. After 1962, the FDA had to act on all submissions, giving its staff and advisory committees more responsibility for policy decisions. Congress also required the FDA to evaluate drugs not only for safety but also for efficacy, although efficacy had not been at issue with thalidomide.

The entire turn of events demonstrates how powerful the symbolic role of the nightmare case can be in implementing public policy. Sustaining the drug regulatory enterprise from 1962 to the AIDS crisis was the image of Kelsey single-handedly saving the public from a greater thalidomide tragedy by saying no to a drug release (Figure 1).

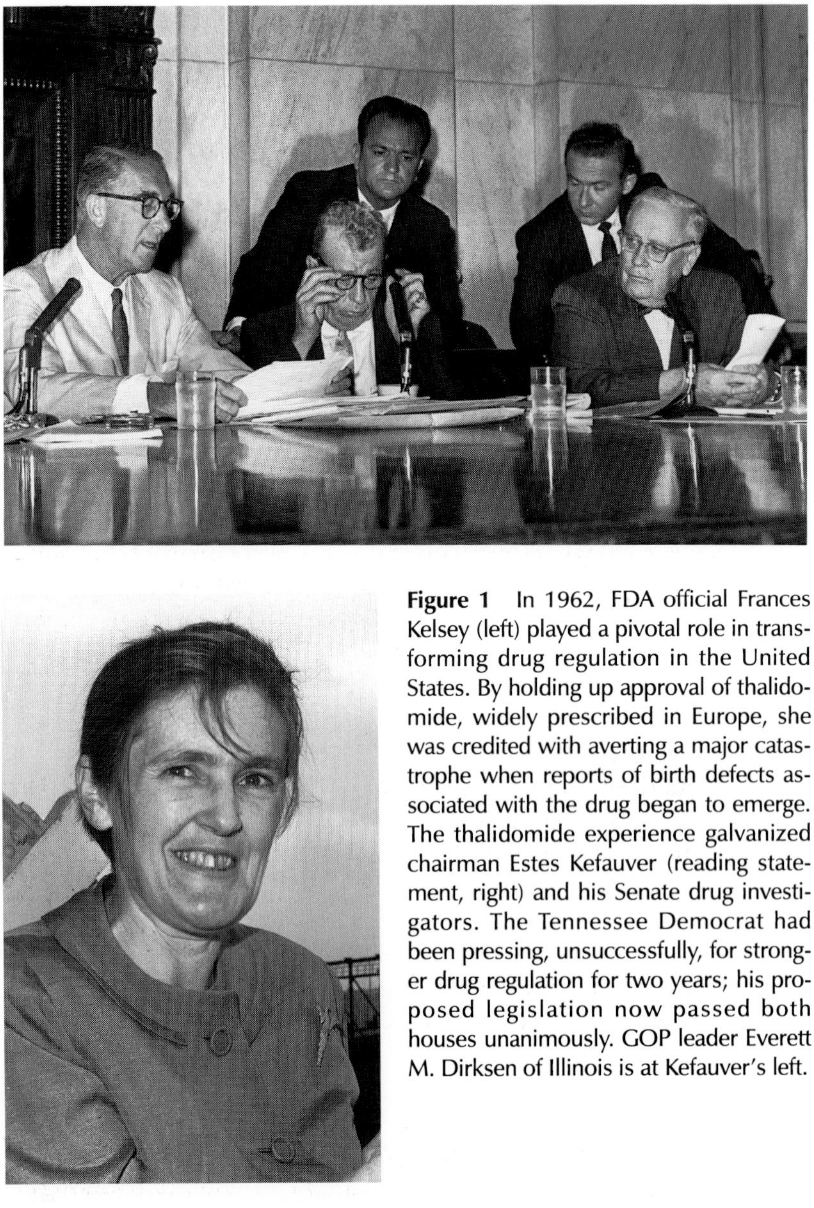

Figure 1 In 1962, FDA official Frances Kelsey (left) played a pivotal role in transforming drug regulation in the United States. By holding up approval of thalidomide, widely prescribed in Europe, she was credited with averting a major catastrophe when reports of birth defects associated with the drug began to emerge. The thalidomide experience galvanized chairman Estes Kefauver (reading statement, right) and his Senate drug investigators. The Tennessee Democrat had been pressing, unsuccessfully, for stronger drug regulation for two years; his proposed legislation now passed both houses unanimously. GOP leader Everett M. Dirksen of Illinois is at Kefauver's left.

Human Experiments

The regulatory authority over the use of human subjects for biomedical research followed a similar and overlapping course. The critical moment came in 1966, when the *New England Journal of Medicine* published an analysis by Henry Beecher, of Harvard Medical School, on "Ethics and Clinical Research." At its core were capsule descriptions of research by 22 investigators and their colleagues who risked "the health or the life of their subjects" without informing them of the dangers or obtaining permission.

Such research included the purposeful withholding of penicillin from U.S. servicemen with streptococcal infections in order to study alternative means of preventing complications. The men were unaware that they were part of an experiment, let alone at risk for rheumatic fever (which a number of them contracted). Children at Willowbrook Hospital, a New York State institution for the retarded on Staten Island, were fed live hepatitis virus vaccine in a study designed to develop effective immunization. Investigators injected live cancer cells into elderly and senile patients at a chronic disease hospital to study the body's immunologic responses. Other investigators inserted needles into the left atrium of subjects with cardiac disease to study heart function.

The *New England Journal* article touched off an outcry for reform that affected Congress and other federal agencies. The solution was to establish a collective mechanism for review of human experimentation. Individual researchers now had to obtain approval of their peers—as well as that of representatives of the wider community—before they could conduct any experiment involving humans. By the mid-1970s, the National Institutes of Health (and the Public Health Service) had in place a system whereby institutional review boards were required to evaluate all such protocols submitted for federal funding to make certain that dangers did not outweigh projected benefits and that subjects had been informed of all significant aspects of the research and had given informed consent.

Along with these regulations came a series of rules to protect the most vulnerable subjects—the institutionalized mentally ill and retarded, children, the elderly, and prisoners—making it difficult if not impossible to use them in research. With the NIH-PHS rules in effect, the FDA added the requirement that protocols testing drugs in humans also secure approval from the review boards.

Thus, regulatory procedures were established on the premise that without supervision, drugs that were dangerous might be released and the rights of human subjects might be ignored. The trade-off was to be slower medical advances for more closely monitored ones.

The 'Drug Lag'

In the context of drug review, there were nay-sayers to FDA supervision both in the pharmaceutical industry and among academicians.

The central complaint was that the FDA was too dilatory and overly wary. These opponents argued that the increase in time and costs in securing marketing approval for a drug—from a couple of years and a few million dollars in 1960, before the Kefauver amendments, to an average of 10 years and nearly $100 million in the 1970s—clearly undercut industry incentives for drug development. They insisted that useful agents were often marketed first in Europe, where drug innovation did not have to confront so many administrative barriers.

Significantly, even the critics of the FDA did not challenge the hierarchical control over testing new drug therapies. They, too, insisted on randomized clinical trials to evaluate efficacy before approval.

The most extraordinary fact about the drug testing regulatory process was that it ran counter to the trends that swept over U.S. medicine in the 1960s and 1970s. Just when patients secured greater autonomy—the right to know a diagnosis, to accept or refuse treatment—the experts at the FDA and review boards controlled the right to regulate new drugs and research protocols. In a period when individual liberties were increasingly respected, this heavy paternalism flourished until the challenge of the 1980s.

Attack on Drug Control

The AIDS epidemic has generated a sustained attack on the basic premises and structure of drug regulation and human research. Advocates for the gay community and AIDS patients have reacted with anger and urgency (Figure 2)—and well they might. They assail the FDA for intransigence in the face of crisis, for taking too long to develop and approve new agents, and for not making potential agents accessible to patients.

As the critics see it, whereas a handful of cases of legionnaires' disease and a few poisoned Tylenol capsules were the scientific equivalent of a five-alarm fire, AIDS initially evoked only a business-as-usual response. Bitterly, these critics imply that gay lives did not matter, and they were unwilling to accept the concept that some lives might have to be sacrificed now to secure better health for later generations.

A coalition of AIDS activists advanced positions in fundamental opposition to those that had dominated the earlier debate. The result was a consumerist approach to medicine and a powerful critique of the drug approval system. If government and the pharmaceutical industry were too slow in developing new therapies, then the AIDS community must organize itself to track down every therapeutic possibility, no matter where in the world it might appear, and then do everything possible to make that drug accessible to its members. Patients with AIDS and their advocates reject the paternalism and risk-averse attitudes of the FDA–review board establishment. And they reject the view that the vulnerable and easily exploited in society need protection from the risks of participation in experimental protocols. From their perspective, experimentation is

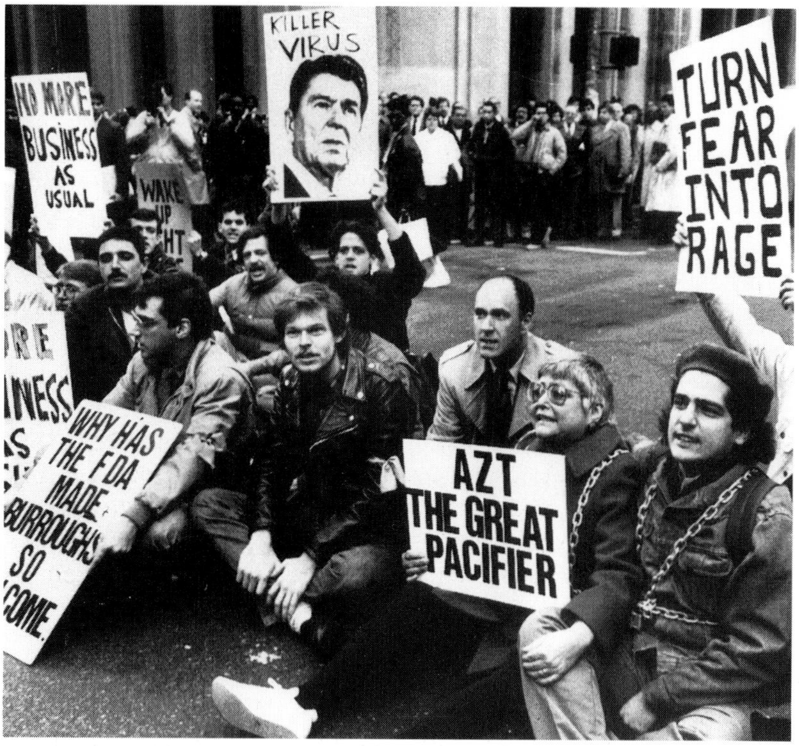
KILLER VIRUS
NO MORE BUSINESS AS USUAL
TURN FEAR INTO RAGE
WHY HAS THE FDA MADE BURROUGHS SO
AZT THE GREAT PACIFIER

Figure 2 Enraged over FDA delays in offering experimental drugs to AIDS patients, gay protestors staged a sit-down demonstration at Broadway and Wall Street in New York in 1987. Several demonstrators were carried away by police.

not a burden but a form of treatment, which should be available to all patients, including even prisoners.

AIDS activists want the FDA to be proactive, not reactive. Their position is that in an epidemic, the agency is obligated to search out any and all possible therapies and, if necessary, sponsor trials to determine a drug's effectiveness and then publicize the results widely. Moreover, in light of the deadly nature of HIV disease, government should not use its authority to restrict experimental treatment to half the patients enrolled in placebo-controlled studies.

It is astonishing that the AIDS critique, especially in its rejection of paternalism, has aligned its advocates with the champions of deregulation in business and with the administration in Washington. Both tend to attribute the failure of conventional medicine to offer better therapy for AIDS to the politics and economics of drug review. Rescind the Kefauver amendment requiring the FDA to measure drug efficacy, declared an editorial in the *Wall Street Journal* (July 14, 1988), and "this single step would help AIDS patients more than any other measure currently being discussed.... In the midst of a medical crisis such as this, where does it say in the Hippocratic oath that patients have to accept a 1962 efficacy rule that forces half of them in these trials to accept a placebo?"

The *Journal* reiterated the theme a few months later. On the occasion of an AIDS protest against government drug regulation (which included lying-in outside FDA headquarters with tombstones reading "I died for the sins of the FDA" and "I got the placebo"), the editorial commented that "it has become a battle between people who have all the time in the world and people who have little time left in their lives."

In fact, much of the AIDS critique of the FDA parallels the long-standing position of the pharmaceutical industry on the drug review process. Government must act faster to approve experimental drugs by requiring less evidence of the drug's efficacy before marketing and let consumers and their physicians decide what greater risks are acceptable. When death is the alternative, the principal job is to find new therapies. There is an incredible irony in all of this. Sick gay men, abandoned by a president who refused publicly to acknowledge their disease on all but one occasion, provided the shock troops to move forward a deregulatory drug control program.

Treating with Investigational Drugs

How then has the AIDS epidemic reshaped drug review practices and law? We will first examine the ways in which the FDA has eased its usual requirements on drug testing to speed approval of experimental drugs, then turn to the thrust to make the FDA more proactive, note the new FDA import policy on drugs, and finally review the parallel track initiative.

In all of these instances, an ongoing and extraordinary effort is being made to address conflicting demands—to respond to the felt needs of the AIDS community amid political pressures, but without abandoning the principles of sound science. Whether this will be sufficient to the crisis and produce a stable and workable drug policy raises complicated medical and ethical questions, and there are no clear answers.

In response to the AIDS advocates, the FDA issued regulations in 1987 that allow treatment with investigational new drugs. These treatment INDs must be under evaluation in controlled trials or the subject of completed trials awaiting analysis; hence, by definition they are of uncertain safety and efficacy. Experimental drugs have been used before in compassionate procedures: Drugs to correct severe cardiac arrhythmias were made widely available in this way before official FDA approval. Now, in the AIDS epidemic, the FDA has codified policy to make INDs available to desperately ill patients before approval of the drugs for full marketing.

Under the AIDS-motivated rules, designated physicians may use INDs for treating patients with immediately life-threatening or other serious disease if no comparable or satisfactory alternative exists. In the regulation, "immediately life threatening" is defined as disease in which there is "reasonable likelihood that death will occur within a matter of months or in which premature death is likely without early treatment." Before treatment INDs can be used, informed consent must be obtained from patients and the local institution's review board must be consulted.

The key question is what standard the FDA will apply in deciding whether to permit treatment INDs. Some observers wonder whether the rules are too permissive. For drugs intended to treat life-threatening disease, treatment INDs are made available if there are enough data to make a reasonable judgment that the drug may be effective and will not expose patients to unreasonable risk. With promising test results, and no sign of major toxicity, the FDA commissioner has no legal right to restrain marketing.

The manufacturer's incentive is the right to sell the investigational drugs. There may be no advertising, no major commercial sale. But practically speaking, advertising may be irrelevant if informed patient groups are prepared instantly to publicize any therapeutic advances, and the government itself is pledged to keep consumers informed about potential AIDS therapies. The price that may be charged for the drug is limited to cost recovery for research, production, and distribution. In turn, charging for an investigational drug permits the FDA to examine accounting records.

A foreseeable problem will be the readiness of third-party payers to reimburse those who purchase the drugs. For years the FDA's stringent requirements on proof of new drug efficacy have served insurance carriers as a shield to resist reimbursement for experimental therapies. Now that the FDA is releasing drugs without any stamp of safety and efficacy, the third-party payers face the issue of reimbursement for an experimental treatment. Under pressure from AIDS groups, several carriers have agreed to pay before the drug has final approval.

The investigational drug uses, with the exceptions noted, still come under the umbrella of the older regulatory system. The new track coexists with the traditional one. The rules strongly caution that the new protocol will be restricted to drugs that are already undergoing controlled clinical trials, while the sponsors are actively pursuing full marketing approval.

But how will trials be performed if patients can buy the investigational drug? Clearly, they would have no incentive to agree to random assignment in a double-blind protocol. One solution, not a pretty one, is a return to the days of ward medicine. In its updated version, the more affluent patients will have early access to promising therapy, while those who cannot afford to pay will be relegated to clinical trials.

Ethics may intervene in the form of some insurance coverage for the poor, but the clinical trial process may well languish for want of adequate enrollment. If that occurs, will the FDA remove a treatment IND from the market even though clinicians are enthusiastic about its effectiveness? That seems very unlikely, although lack of data from trials will foreclose definitive assessment of the drug's efficacy.

Toward a Proactive FDA

Even as such questions remain open, the FDA has moved on other fronts. FDA regulations in effect since October 1988 commit the agency to assist pharmaceutical sponsors in developing drugs for life-threatening and serious diseases. As a result, the federal government will increasingly participate in deciding what drugs are tested and how.

The central thrust of the October 1988 regulations is to involve the FDA in clinical trial planning. With such involvement, the expectation is that shorter, better-planned trials will result (or perhaps that the FDA will be less likely to challenge the adequacy of trials that it helped design in the first place). When drug sponsors want to test a new product, they may confer with FDA officials early in drug development on the design of necessary preclinical and clinical studies. Involvement of the FDA in the process of clinical study design may thus neutralize the adversarial posture between the regulators and the regulated.

The regulations acknowledge that a faster review process will inevitably entail unresolved potential problems. Accordingly, a subtle shift in drug approval standards is incorporated. The 1962 statute required that drugs be proved safe and effective. Now, for products to treat life-threatening or debilitating illnesses, the FDA proposed to grant approval on the basis of medical risk-benefit ratios. In effect, if the benefits appear to be substantial, the FDA will permit a drug to be marketed even though some safety parameters are still unknown. It will then seek to determine the precise range of drug effects and dangers in postmarketing studies.

The Import Policy

Probably the greatest concession to AIDS activism has been the FDA's reversal on importation of drugs. Unlike the other innovations we have reviewed, this one is not embodied in statutes or regulations. It was announced at a 1988 National Lesbian and Gay Health Conference and AIDS Forum by then FDA commissioner Frank E. Young (Figure 3), who spoke about the ways in which the FDA's enforcement authority would henceforth be exercised.

The new import policy derived directly from the fight by AIDS patients for access to dextran sulfate, which is obtainable only from abroad. The FDA would now permit anyone—not just AIDS patients—to import small quantities of such an unapproved drug. The imported drugs may not be for commercial sale; they are limited to personal use by the patient, who must supply the name of a physician who will be providing treatment. If these conditions are met, the patient may either personally bring such drugs across U.S. borders or use the mails to do so.

This was a bold departure from the FDA's past insistence on its legal duty to enforce prohibitions against introducing unproven drugs into U.S. commerce. (Indeed, dextran sulfate was subsequently shown to have *no* clinical efficacy.) The reality was that large numbers of AIDS pa-

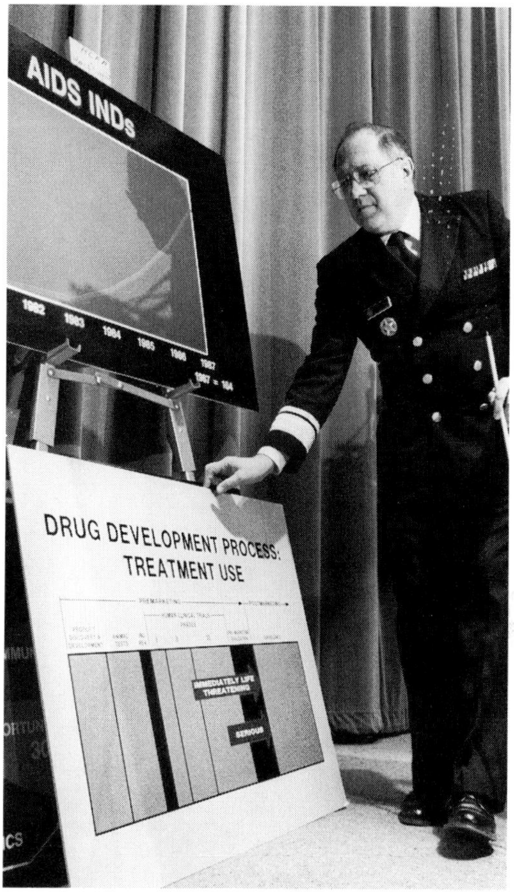

Figure 3 In 1988, FDA Commissioner Frank Young announced a new import policy for unapproved drugs from abroad—an important departure from the agency's past insistence on strict embargo. In truth, AIDS patients and those infected with HIV were already bringing in experimental drugs.

tients and those infected with HIV were already bringing in experimental drugs from Mexico, Europe, and Japan. At the least, the new import policy added to that reality some supervision by physicians.

Still, the change stunned some AIDS researchers, who pointed out that if government allows unproven drugs to circulate freely, rigorous drug testing will be far more difficult to accomplish. If patients can take a variety of drugs in unknown combinations, it may be impossible to sort out the subtle signs of efficacy or toxicity. In the long run, the policy may only prolong the time needed to develop new AIDS drugs while opening the doors, as has been said, to purveyors of snake oil. Other researchers, however, are more confident that the clinical trial process can still be maintained.

Parallel Tracking

The parallel track program is another product of the pressures for new AIDS treatment. Its content was extensively discussed by government and patient advocacy groups between July 1989 and May 1990. Understandably, these groups had different agendas. Some saw the parallel track as an opportunity to collect more data, others as one to facilitate provision of care. The basic question, however, was how to expand access to new drugs beyond that permitted by the treatment IND. After all, treatment IND regulations for drugs directed at life-threatening diseases require only a "may help and no proof of harm" standard. What reasonable standard for clinical use could be more permissive than that a drug *may* help?

On May 21, 1990, the Public Health Service issued a notice of proposed policy that represented the first regulatory embodiment of the parallel track concept. It is not accidental that this proposal came from the PHS and not the FDA, because it amounts, at least in part, to an about-face on the liberalized treatment IND and drug import policies previously promulgated by the FDA.

The proposed PHS policy gives patients with AIDS and HIV-related diseases access to promising investigational drugs. However, the only patients eligible are 1) those unable to take standard therapy, 2) those in whom such therapy is no longer effective, and 3) those who cannot participate in the relevant clinical trials. Compared with treatment IND criteria, this clearly restricts the number of patients with access. Indeed, what is striking about the proposed PHS policy is its insistence that clinical trials come first and that the parallel track may not delay or compromise that process.

Moreover, the new policy states that a treatment IND *may* be granted when sufficient data are available suggesting a drug's possible efficacy without unreasonable risks. Such language makes the treatment IND discretionary rather than mandatory. In effect, the "may help" standard is to be read narrowly in order to accommodate a parallel track. On the other hand, the proposed policy statement also says that expanded-availability protocols *might* be approved for promising investigational drugs when the evidence of efficacy is less than that generally required for treatment INDs. Given the treatment IND standard that a drug need only possibly be effective, however, it is difficult to imagine a lower standard that would be consistent with any scientific evidence whatsoever.

In all of this—from the treatment IND, to drug importation, to the parallel track and beyond—it is evident that the AIDS advocates have largely succeeded in doing what earlier critics were unable to do: taking more decisions out of the hands of government and the research establishment and ceding them to patients and their physicians. In the ultimate calculation of risks and benefits, those coping with the deadly progress of HIV infection should decide what risks to take.

From another view, the changes in public policy represent a strategic retreat on the part of the federal regulators. The FDA would make new rules for new drugs, but would safeguard the clinical trial process to learn what works best. But is the clinical trial the exclusive key to knowledge? Given a disease that may be uniformly fatal, should drug testing use placebo controls?

Leaders in the AIDS community, having had tangible successes at the

FDA on drug regulation, are moving on to the next phase. They will be attempting to shift funds allocated for research to AIDS. However, they will then be competing with other disease groups who, perhaps inspired by the example of AIDS advocates, can be expected to launch parallel assaults on what they perceive as paternalistic regulation.

SELECTED READING

Edgar H, Rothman DJ: New rules for new drugs: The challenge of AIDS to the regulatory process. Milbank Q 68 (suppl 1): 111, 1990

Rothman DJ, Edgar H: Drug approval and AIDS: Benefits for the elderly. Health Aff (Millwood) 9: 123, 1990

Lasagna L: Congress, the FDA, and the new drug development: Before and after 1962. Perspect Biol Med 32: 322, 1989

Rothman DJ: Ethics and human experimentation: Henry Beecher revisited. N Engl J Med 317: 1195, 1987

Rothman DJ: Strangers at the Bedside: A History of How Law and Bioethics Transformed Medical Decision Making. Basic Books, New York, 1991

Delaney M: The case for patient access to experimental therapy. J Infect Dis 159: 416, 1989

Fox P: From senility to Alzheimer's disease: The rise of the Alzheimer's disease movement. Milbank Q 67: 58, 1989

Kessler D: The regulation of investigational drugs. N Engl J Med 320: 281, 1989

Index

Note: Numerals in *italics* indicate a figure; "t" following a page number indicates a table.

COLS
WRIGHT STATE UNIVERSITY
HEALTH SCIENCES LIBRARY
0 00 13 06741 27 1

WD 308 A00843 1993

AIDS

The Fordham Library

WRIGHT STATE

Wright State University
Dayton, Ohio 45435

DEMCO